Praise for *A Race j*

"Inspiring, medically sound, and beautifully written. I would like to share this book with all of my patients and friends. Hearing the message from Ruth's perspective makes for a heart-warming journey and a solid prescription for optimum well being."—**Neal D. Barnard**, M.D., author, *Eat Right, Live Longer* and *Foods That Fight Pain*

"Ruth's story of surviving breast cancer, adopting a plant-based diet and becoming a winning world class triathlete is both exhilarating and terrifying. With discipline, exuberance and resilience, Ruth faced each challenge including two near-fatal highway collisions and an alarming medical setback. Her life-affirming attitude shines through her whole remarkable story from sickness to health, from tragedy to triumph. What an inspiration for all!"—**Dorothy Greet**, educator, speaker, author of *Go Veg With Class*, www.GoVegWithClass.com

"*A Race for Life* is more than an athlete's memoir; it's a testament to the human spirit's capacity to overcome adversity and a practical guide for anyone looking to enhance their health and vitality naturally. Ruth Heidrich, alongside experts in medicine, coaching, and nutrition, provides compelling evidence that a life of exceptional wellness is achievable for all of us. Her fascinating story is a beacon of hope and a blueprint for a healthier, more fulfilling life, proving that with the right mix of discipline, knowledge, and spirit, the battle against even the most daunting challenges can be won."—**Chef AJ**, former television host, executive pastry chef, and author

"*A Race for Life* is an inspiring story by a remarkable woman. Dr. Ruth is a portrait in courage and perseverance, serving as an example of how we can face and overcome obstacles, whatever they may be, on our life journey. Her book is especially valuable for older readers! Empowered with knowledge of the health benefits of the vegan lifestyle, we can give ourselves the best chance to flourish in our advanced age with good health, vitality, mental acuity, and purpose."
—**Dr. Joanne Kong**, editor, *Vegan Voices: Essays by Inspiring Changemakers*

"Dr. Ruth Heidrich's friendship, guidance, and wisdom I've valued greatly since reaching out to her in early December 2010. A thyroid cancer diagnosis in the Fall of '04 shook me hard at age 42 in my 'prime;' with a wonderful wife, life and three beautiful young daughters. Two surgeries and one heavy dose of radiated iodine left me with no detectable thyroid tissue in early '05, and a focus on what I could do going forward to minimize risk of any type of cancer diagnosis. The medical community seemed clueless as to why the cancer happened and what specifically I could do better, aside from vague suggestions about eating well and resting. Annual follow up scans left a sense of persistent fear.

By Fall of '09, I'd run my first marathon after some modest diet improvements, fasting and weight loss. After a few failed attempts at getting off my prescribed statins, in frustration I reached out to Ruth.

I'd learned of Ruth's inspirational story while reading the best seller, *Born to Run*, in early 2010 and reached out to her directly. When the student is ready, the teacher will come. I was ready and so was Ruth.

Ruth was gracious, brilliant, and patient with my questions that week. Dec. 10th is now my 'veganversary.' I'm happy and proud to be into a 14th year 100% plant powered. The positive changes have gone way beyond expectations. Within about three months I was able to flush my statins down for good. By early June of '11 I ran a first ultramarathon and have not let up since. I've lost track of how many 50K races completed. 100-mile foot races are my primary goal, with 27 official finishes thus far. My vision improved and amazing people came into my life. The unintended positive consequences continue to go on and on. I pay it forward and often share Ruth's true story, even with fellow runners during 100-mile races.

Ruth's great gift to me was the shift from fear of chronic disease to joy, adventure, and gratitude. I like to say 'ease' requires a great deal of energy, but let's strive to live with 'ease' vs. disease. I think of this as an upward spiral that requires constant awareness. Ruth helped lead me to a focus on desires vs. concerns.

Read *A Race for Life* and her other books. I'll never forget Ruth hand delivering three copies of *Lifelong Running*. She ran them to me in her local Hawaii marathon shirt, while visiting Wright Patterson Air Force Base.

Life's most important decisions should include some thought about who we should listen to. I love influencers with decades of experience, expertise, evidence, and passion. Ruth offers that and more."—**Randy Kreill**, BRFT-VGN-RNNR

"This is the book I wished I'd had back when I was 40. It is so inspiring to read about what Ruth Heidrich went through to become a Stage 4 breast cancer survivor. As if that weren't enough, she covers what it takes to be an Ironman triathlete, mentally as well as physically. It would be a great gift for any woman, athlete or not."—**Karina Lok**, senior vegan runner

"Ruth's wisdom is well-founded in science as well as her own personal experience. This book—chock-full of good information—is good reading as well. For those wanting to be well and fit, read *A Race for Life*."—**Jim Mason**, author, *An Unnatural Order*

"Ruth Heidrich serves as an inspiration for every woman fighting for her life and dignity. Given the right foods and exercise she proves the human body is its own greatest healer. Don't miss this opportunity to take charge of your life." —**John McDougall**, M.D., author, *McDougall Program for Women*

"Everyone needs to read this book! It's such a compelling story of hope and healing! You can't put the book down until you are finished! Dr. Ruth is such an inspiration for life. This book is great!"—**Cindy Meuse**, a dedicated fan

"A passionate testimonial by an extraordinary woman who turned tragedy to triumph through vigorous exercise and refined diet. Ruth Heidrich's experiences point to the potential in all of us when we turn knowledge to action, to create healthier, more vibrant lives."—**Dan Millman**, author, *Way of the Peaceful Warrior* and *Body Mind Mastery*

"Dr. Ruth Heidrich is a fear annihilator. She's faced head-on the two greatest fears that women have—breast cancer and growing old—and shows that it's possible to overcome the former and transform the latter. Surely everyone's story is different, but in reading hers, we can collect tools to apply to our own, along with inspiration, courage, and a role model bar none."—**Victoria Moran**, author, *The Love-Powered Diet* and *Age Like a Yogi*

"Ruth Heidrich is a trailblazer in every way . . . she had breast cancer but declined the standard treatment, defying the advice of the medical establishment at the time, and she has come out victorious as a more than 40-year survivor of breast cancer and an Iron Woman athlete! She was doing lifestyle medicine before it even existed! In this book, Ruth tells us about her journey and how she modified her lifestyle for optimum health. You can follow her lead, as she lays it out step by step in this book and optimize your health as well! She continues to be an inspiration for us all."—**Dr. Grace Chen O'Neil**, MD, FACEP

"*A Race for Life* was the first book I published at Lantern, back in 2000, and like Ruth herself, it remains an evergreen example of tenacity, resilience, passion, and maximizing your potential. *A Race for Life* began Lantern's (and my own running) journey, and I'm delighted that we're all still going strong!"—**Martin Rowe**, editor, *Running, Eating, Thinking: A Vegan Anthology* and Executive Director of Culture & Animals Foundation

"I knew and admired Ruth Heidrich long before I ever met her. When I was a mom of a young child, I happened to read her book *A Race for Life*. Her story of overcoming a usually fatal diagnosis of metastatic cancer, and then being able to compete successfully in some of the most grueling athletic competitions in the world electrified me. She inspired me so much that I bought more copies of her book, as well as the video of A Race for Life, and gave them away to others also facing the challenge of cancer, whether for themselves or for their loved ones.

Little did I know that one day, I would also come to know Ruth as a dear friend, and as a colleague in our volunteer efforts with the Vegan Society of Hawaii, of which she has been a founding member since it began in 1990 as the Vegetarian Society of Honolulu and later, as the Vegetarian Society of Hawaii. Ruth is, in fact, a past president of VSH, a nonprofit, all-volunteer organization whose mission is to promote human health, animal rights, and protection of the environment by means of whole food, plant-based vegan education.

Now, over four decades since what could have been a totally dispiriting and life-ending illness, and since she met Dr. John McDougall, also a hero to me, who gave this brilliant and tenacious mind of hers the factual tools she needed to build a peaceful arsenal against one of the health scourges of our time, she's come out with an updated version of her milestone book and story that has become the shot heard 'round the world,' as she continues to inspire and inform yet another generation!"—**Lorraine Sakaguchi**, President of Vegan Society of Hawaii

"For years now, both medical and physical evidence has pointed to diet, exercise, and emotional well-being as contributing in great measure to the prevention of cancer, as well as to some rather miraculous remissions or, in some cases, outright cures.

Ruth Heidrich tells a fascinating story of her progression from a woman devastated by the thought of losing her breasts—and quite possibly her life—because of cancer to an internationally recognized athlete.

Ruth's story needs to be told—not to glorify her athletic prowess, which is a story in itself, but to demonstrate that there is a mix of diet, exercise, and mental conditioning that anyone of us can use to fight the invasion of disease and depression in a natural way.

Along with medical professionals, coaches, and nutritionists who are gathering evidence for our future benefit, people like Ruth Heidrich are at the forefront, proving that the way to a healthier, happier life free of disease starts here, today."—**Terry Shintani**, MD, JD, MPH, Author of *Eat More, Weigh Less*; *The Hawaii Diet*; *The Peace Diet*; *The Good Carbohydrate Revolution*; and *Lose Weight While You Sleep*

"Dr. Ruth and her books are my 'go-to' for answers to my questions about diet and exercise! She keeps so up to date in the health and fitness field, so deluged with information (often misinformation), determining what is correct and pertinent and then generously informs everyone with her books, etc. Her determination to make her life better inspires and encourages those of us not quite as determined and willing! She does this with grace, kindness, and acceptance, making me want to be better. Endless kudos and praise to this great lady and her new highly readable and practical book—I recommend it to anyone who can read and wishes to get better!"—**Lynne Stahl**, 83-year young marathoner

"This inspiring story led me to a 30+ year friendship with Ruth Heidrich who taught me many things including "You can learn to like what's good for you."—**Lorenn Walker**, JD, MPH, author, *Aging With Strength*

A RACE FOR LIFE

A Diet and Exercise Program
for Super-Fitness and Reversing
the Aging Process

*The amazing story of how one woman survived
breast cancer to take on the toughest races in the world*

Ruth E. Heidrich, PhD

Lantern Publishing & Media ● Woodstock & Brooklyn, NY

2024
Lantern Publishing & Media
PO Box 1350
Woodstock, NY 12498
www.lanternpm.org

Cover design by Pauline Lafosse

Printed in the United States of America

Library of Congress Cataloging-in-Publication Data

Names: Heidrich, Ruth, author.
Title: A race for life : a diet and exercise program for superfitness and reversing the aging process / Ruth E. Heidrich.
Description: [Revised edition] | Brooklyn, NY : Lantern Publishing & Media, 2024. | "This title was previously published by Booklight Inc. (DBA Lantern Books)." | Includes bibliographical references.
Identifiers: LCCN 2023046291 (print) | LCCN 2023046292 (ebook) | ISBN 9781590567104 (paperback) | ISBN 9781590567111 (epub)
Subjects: LCSH: Health. | Physical fitness. | Nutrition. | Heidrich, Ruth—Health. | Breast—Cancer—Patients—Hawaii—Biography. | BISAC: HEALTH & FITNESS / Diet & Nutrition / General | SELF-HELP / Motivational & Inspirational
Classification: LCC RA776 .H465 2024 (print) | LCC RA776 (ebook) | DDC 613—dc23/eng/20240126
LC record available at https://lccn.loc.gov/2023046291
LC ebook record available at https://lccn.loc.gov/2023046292

Contents

This book is dedicated to all who are interested in improving the quality and length of their lives and who care about animals and the environment. May you forever avoid the scourge of heart disease, cancer, stroke, diabetes, arthritis, osteoporosis, hypertension, obesity, autoimmune diseases, dementia, and all the other diseases influenced one way or another by diet and exercise.

Acknowledgments

Writing this book has turned out to be an incredible adventure. I could never have done it without the support of some wonderful people.

First, I owe a huge debt of gratitude to Kenneth Cooper, MD, who published his ground-breaking book *Aerobics* way back in 1968. At that time, I happened to be at a newsstand looking for something to read on a long flight back home. I noticed a word I'd never seen before since Dr. Cooper had just coined it. Curious as to what it meant, I bought the book and read the whole thing on that flight. I discovered the many benefits of aerobic-type exercise, which uses the major muscle groups to increase your lungs' capacity to process oxygen, which is why Dr. Cooper titled his book with this new word. *Aerobics* covers running, walking, cycling, swimming, and any activity that increases your heart rate and makes you anaerobic. Thank you, Dr. Cooper!

My second huge debt of gratitude is to John A. McDougall, MD, the physician who turned my life around by educating me about my newly diagnosed cancer and following my progress, me being a volunteer subject in his breast cancer research. Dr. McDougall was the first to suggest that I write a book about what I learned on this medical journey, saying that it would be of value to others. He believed in me enough to almost literally take me by the hand to a computer store where he showed me the wonders of computers and word processing. He'd periodically check up on me, assuring me that "it's easy once you get started." Dr. McDougall was right. Looking back from my current vantage point, I see that writing this book was easy, though it had seemed nearly impossible at the beginning. Thank you, Dr. McDougall!

Next, the late John Kay came into my life. He'd read my story in the Hawaii publication *Midweek*. After introducing himself to me, he asked if I'd ever thought about writing a book. I told him that, by chance, Dr. McDougall had suggested it and I'd just started seriously considering it. He volunteered to help, and help he did. Each week, we met for him to review the previous week's painful efforts. (Writing is easy: you just sit down at the keyboard and open a vein and hope the words pour out!) He critiqued my writing, patted me on the back, and sent me off to write some more.

As I increased my exercise, I ran into resistance from people—even doctors—who thought that I, as a cancer patient, should be "taking it easy and not stressing my body so much." Thankfully, my track coach, Johnny Faerber, supported me in my efforts to run faster and, likewise, my distance coach, Max Telford, in my efforts to run farther. As my "unorthodox" medical program gained more attention, I started to get some publicity. This led to an invitation for me to fly to Hollywood for an appearance on the nationally televised program *Hour Magazine*, hosted by Gary Collins. I got to tell the show's large audience about Dr. Cooper and how he launched me on my running career, about Dr. McDougall and how his dietary guidance altered my life forever, enabling me to become the very first vegan, male or female, and cancer patient to complete an Ironman triathlon back in 1983.

Terry Shintani, MD, entered the scene by giving me the opportunity to be co-host of a weekly, two-hour radio talk show called *Nutrition and You*, on which, for my weekly "Fitness Report," I covered the latest research on the many benefits of daily, effective exercise. Our show came on every Sunday night for well over ten years until that radio station went off the air. Working with Dr. Shintani has been invaluable: as both a physician and a friend, he has given me much support. In addition, we've had some fabulous guests on our show; I have learned a lot from and really owe Bonnie Choy, RN, the late Bill Harris, MD, the late Carl Weisbrod, PhD, Katie Paine, and a host of others.

I owe a lot to another group of people, my physical therapists. They have my greatest respect for what they know and teach. After I was hit by a truck twice while training on my bike, sustaining devastating injuries including multifocal fractures (fractures on both sides of my body) and a concussion, they were highly instrumental in getting me back on the road. There were a number of physical therapists of different specialties who taught me knowledge of my anatomy and techniques that helped me move better, feel better, and perform better. I would like them all to know that I continue to practice those routines to this day as my form of maintenance after rehab. I believe physical therapy should continue throughout life and is especially important as we age.

I've also been given the opportunity to give presentations on diet and exercise to audiences all over the world. I've shared a platform with notables such as T. Colin Campbell, PhD, Neal Barnard, MD, Caldwell Esselstyn, MD, Michael Klaper, MD, and Brenda Davis, RD, not only in the US but also in Thailand, Scotland, Canada, and Singapore. I was actually on my way to Istanbul to give a talk when 9/11 struck, leaving me stranded in London for a week. The Istanbul conference got canceled, as were all my flights, as a result of the shocking and devastating turn of events.

Lastly, I am grateful for having been one of the "stars" of the groundbreaking documentary *Forks over Knives*. As I was traveling a lot, people in different places—from Florida to Alaska and everywhere in between—recognized me and enthusiastically told me how watching it had changed their lives forever!

And there are countless more people who continue to support and inspire me on this journey that is far from over.

FOREWORD

Even though Ruth Heidrich has accomplished feats that most of us don't even dream of, she might be the most relatable author I have ever read. A good storyteller, who makes you want to join her as a friend and confidant. Her internal thoughts mirrored what I imagine my own might be in her shoes.

A Race for Life was already a book I had been recommending to others for many years. Not just those facing a cancer diagnosis, but anyone looking for inspiration to live more healthfully. However, this updated edition has added importance (post COVID) for everyone. Our medical system is far more broke than any of us imagined possible back when Ruth went through her cancer treatment. Regulatory agencies, public health officials, medical boards, and medical journal publishers now act like full partners with industry, rather than gatekeepers intent on protecting us from its excesses.

In her new chapter 18, she shares a most profound insight: "What I did not know at the time were the questions that I should have asked: Where was the evidence that silicone implants are safe?" Everyone would be well advised to globalize this insight to *everything* any medical "expert" advises.

It matters more now than any other time in our lives to apply deep critical thinking to keeping ourselves healthy enough that we avoid falling into the grip of the dysfunctional modern medical system . . . and this book will help you to do just that.

JoAnn Farb
Former microbiologist, author, health educator,
and blogger at JoAnnFarb.com

INTRODUCTION

Diagnosis

I could not believe what I'd just heard. The words "infiltrating ductal carcinoma" shocked, terrified, and then numbed me. It was cancer! That lump that had just been cut out of my breast was cancer! As the impact of this potential death sentence began to sink in, a wild and uncontrollable panic seized me. "Oh, no!" I cried. "Oh, no, no." The devastating words of that diagnosis of cancer echoed in my head as I fought back dizziness and nausea. I felt as if I were in some horrible nightmare from which I was about to awaken.

Just minutes before, while waiting to hear the results of the biopsy from the pathology lab, I had been so sure—in fact, certain—from the two previous biopsies that the offending growth had to be benign. I kept telling myself to quit worrying, that everything was going to be just fine—just like it had always been every other time in my life when tragedy had loomed. Hadn't I always done everything I was supposed to do? As the reality sank in, I felt totally alone. No one heard my silent screams. "This can't be happening to me!" "This is not fair!" My life had just been turned upside down. Suddenly, my focus was laser-beamed on *cancer*. My obsession was total; all else in my life fell by the wayside.

I had always eaten what I'd been taught in my university class on nutrition (what is, unfortunately, still taught in most of these classes) to be a "well-balanced" diet. Years before, I had sworn off red meat and white bread; I had even started taking the skin off chicken. I had switched to low-fat powdered milk as a good source of calcium for my bones. I had gotten plenty of exercise as a daily runner for fourteen years and, in fact, had even run several marathons. I had had frequent medical check-ups, including regular mammograms, and had religiously examined my breasts every month.

How could this have happened? And why to me? *Things like this happen only in the movies or to other people*, I thought. I'd always led a relatively conventional life, being healthy and successful and always playing by the rules. Some would even say that in the game of life, I'd been dealt a good hand. I was attractive enough to have won a few beauty contests and to have made three appearances in the original TV series *Hawaii Five-0*. As a proud UCLA graduate, I was well educated; as a GS-13 military logistician, I held an engrossing, well-paying job that let me travel to military bases all over the world. All four of my grandparents had lived to their nineties, so I assumed I had some pretty good genes. I had what I thought was a good, solid marriage, with two bright, beautiful, and successful children. My life could not have been better.

But that streak of good luck had just been devastated! Suddenly, my life revolved around a new role, that of "cancer patient." I didn't even know anyone in the same situation as mine, so I asked around to see if anyone knew of anyone else who had breast cancer, but no one did. Obsessed with trying to find out why I'd gotten my diagnosis, I was disheartened when each doctor I asked said that no one knew.

I went to the library and brought home the very few books on cancer there were, one of which said that my type of cancer was "moderately fast-metastasizing," which only added to my anxiety. I kept thinking there had to be a mistake. I decided to get not just one but four "second" opinions. All that yielded was the dashing of any hope that my pathology report had been a misdiagnosis. And still, not one of the doctors could tell me why I had gotten cancer.

So why this avalanche of devastation? To me, my diagnosis was both a life and a death sentence—a "life" sentence because there's still no real cure for breast cancer, and a "death" sentence because breast cancer is a major killer of adult women, at that time striking one out of thirteen American women (although it's now one out of every seven or eight). It also happens to be the number-one killer of women in my age group.

"My God, what do I do now?" I asked the two surgeons who were attending me. "More surgery," the senior surgeon said. "I'd recommend a modified radical mastectomy since the tumor was so large, with no clear margins, so we know we didn't get it all."

I had talked the surgeons into letting me watch that first operation (against their better judgment, according to them), which was an excisional biopsy, meaning that they tried to remove the whole growth. Having been administered only a local anesthetic instead of general anesthesia, I had watched in awe as the surgeon carved a chunk the size of a golf ball out of my right breast. Thinking that the size of the mass must be exaggerated in my mind, I kept trying to diminish it. But sure enough, the pathology report had shown that it was more than five centimeters (or two inches), again, with "no clear margins." No, it was still horribly big no matter how I visualized it.

The type of surgery now recommended to me would remove all the breast tissue that remained after the biopsy, the fascia covering the chest muscles, the skin covering the breast area, and the nipple (leaving no mastectomy flaps), plus the lymph nodes in the axilla (armpit). A lumpectomy was out of the question because there were cancer cells beyond all the margins of the tissue sample. The surgeons told me that after the surgery, there would be tests to determine the spread. As it turned out, three of the tests turned up positive, each with some evidence of the spread of the cancer: a positive bone scan, a liver panel that showed extremely high liver enzymes, plus a chest x-ray that indicated a suspicious lesion in my left lung. It would have taken a lung biopsy to determine whether it was cancerous, but since I'd just undergone surgery, they decided to watch and see if it grew. After six months of watching, they determined that it was not growing and had encapsulated—a very good sign, which they interpreted as my immune system walling it off.

By that time, I was feeling betrayed by my breasts anyway, so they had no problem in getting me to agree to a second mastectomy, telling me that I was at high risk of getting cancer in the other breast. (We now know that's not necessarily true because the intervention of a healthy low-fat, whole-food, plant-based vegan diet stops the excessive estrogen that can both initiate and fuel cancer cells.) Still, after both surgeries, I was given no assurance that my life would be saved, even *with* chemotherapy and radiation. This was because it is the nature of cancerous tumors to immediately start shedding cells and growing their own blood vessels (a process called angiogenesis), which then spread cancer cells to distant parts of the body, most frequently bones, the brain, the lungs, and the liver. So, cutting off my breasts at that point was akin to proverbially closing the barn doors after the horse has escaped. Adding chemotherapy and radiation produced no promise of nonrecurrence either and, in fact, could cause permanent damage to my immune system.

The doctors (there were now three of them in the room) shook their heads in anticipation of my next question. "We don't know if you have three months, three years, or how long," they said. "We just know that it's a type of moderately fast-metastasizing cancer, and we know the possible extent of the spread because of its large size. We certainly don't know why; there's an awful lot we just don't know. . . ."

To add to my anxiety, I recalled that when I had come in earlier that week, the doctor, looking at the plainly visible lump in my breast, had asked with great concern in his voice, "Why did you wait so long to come in?" Instantly panicking, I flew into a rage at the same time.

"What do you mean '*wait so long*'?" I practically screamed. "I was just here three months ago and was told this was only scar tissue from a previous biopsy." I was sputtering by now. "I even had another mammogram at that time, which they assured me was negative."

I calmed myself down, took a deep breath, and said, "I was here six months ago, then again three months ago when I tried to tell them that this 'scar tissue' was growing, but they kept telling me that everything was normal." It was actually three years before that when I had first found that lump, much smaller then, and had been assured that it was "nothing to worry about."

I suddenly realized that the biopsy a year earlier had actually, as they said, just removed scar tissue and so had missed the nearby cancer. Now it might be too late! Having breast cancer was bad enough. Finding out that the cancer had been obviously growing in my breast for at least three years because of the inexperience, ignorance, or arrogance of a doctor was almost more than I could bear.

Enter Angiogenesis and Myokines

What I didn't know at the time of my diagnosis was that there was a fight going on in my body. On one side was angiogenesis, the ability of cancer cells to secrete substances that allow them to form their own blood supply, which is what enables the cancer to spread. On the other were myokines, special proteins that suppress the same cancer's spread and that were produced by my running and exercise. It is angiogenesis that allows a cancerous mass to grow larger than just a few millimeters by supplying the needed oxygen and nutrients. Since my tumor was more than five centimeters, this explained how it had spread to my bones and one of my lungs, causing the horrible bone pain and vague chest pain I was experiencing. I was prescribed a narcotic for the bone pain and nitroglycerin for the chest pain, neither of which helped at all. What I didn't know at the time was that my continued running—the exercising of my skeletal muscles—was producing myokines, proteins that may have been helping fight back the cancer.[1]

Pressing On . . .

"Never mind," he said, "we're going to schedule surgery right away."

My eyes brimming with tears, I was experiencing the worst moment of my life. I wanted to scream, yell, hit out, rage, and vent my fury, and at the same time to just roll over and give up. It was already too late; I might as well die right now! I was engulfed with feelings of total despair and hopelessness.

Hey, wait just a darn minute, I thought. *Hold on! No, I'm* not *ready to roll over and die. I am going to fight to live—fight this death sentence with everything I have.* So how could I afford to get angry at the very people I was counting on to help save my life?

If I had only a short time remaining, I needed to get busy. I had a lot of work to do. Thus began my "race for life."

The Operation: Modified Radical Mastectomy

Unfortunately, detaching me from my breasts wasn't that simple as it entailed fairly extensive surgery. But it wasn't that difficult either. When I checked into the hospital the night before the mastectomy, the nurses who helped me unpack were amazed to see running shorts, singlets, sweat bands, running shoes, socks, and not much else. I hadn't bothered with bras and regular clothing, feeling that I wasn't going to need them. I could see the nurses shaking their heads as they walked out of the room. What they didn't understand was that since I'd been a daily runner for fourteen years at that point, I wasn't about to let this hospital stay interrupt my daily routine any more than absolutely necessary.

It dawned on me that since I was here in the hospital, I could ask to see the mammogram that had just given me the false-negative result. I wanted to see for myself how they could have missed that very large tumor. I asked to see the chief of radiology, who pulled up my mammogram on the screen, and I pointed to exactly where my tumor was. Looking closely with his magnifying glass, he said that there was no sign of the tumor and that my breasts, being somewhat dense, had obviously hidden it. He then added that about one eighth of screening mammograms are false negatives, especially when the breasts are dense.

Getting in One Last Run

On the morning of the surgery, the head nurse walked into my hospital room to administer the pre-operative medication, the drugs routinely given to patients to allay anxiety and relax them. My bed, however, was empty.

"My God," the head nurse said to her aide, as relayed to me by the latter. "She's run away! And here we thought she was taking this so well." I'd been told the pre-op medication would be given to me at 5 a.m., so I'd set my alarm for 4 a.m., crawled out of bed, slipped into my running clothes, tip-toed down the shadowy halls, and escaped into the still-dark hills surrounding the hospital. I covered six miles in what was one of the most satisfying runs ever.

All the fear, tension, stress, anxiety, and even anger seemed to drain away, replaced with a declaration, "Okay, we are going to *war*!" I had this powerful feeling—like I was an army general waging a war on the battlefield that was my chest! The surgeons (all *four* of them now) were colonels on the operating-room front; the nurses were in charge of the mop-up operations; and the rest of the medical support personnel, with their weapons (needles, tubes, drugs) and various areas of expertise, were awaiting their call to arms.

At the end of the sixth mile, I was ready to do battle. I turned back to the hospital and as I approached the entrance, I was shocked to see my surgeon just arriving. He was even more shocked to see me! "What in the world are you doing here?" he asked incredulously. I actually felt pangs of guilt; I knew that they'd never have given me permission to run if I'd asked.

As it turned out, the staff most certainly would *not* have allowed me to run. When you run, you sweat. Sweating causes dehydration. On the day of surgery, you will not have been able to eat or drink anything since midnight, so you tend to be a little dehydrated anyway. Here was a sweaty, thirsty, and dehydrated patient presenting to surgery, as they say. The head nurse was chewed out for not keeping a closer eye on her charge, and the surgeon told the anesthesiologist to pump some extra intravenous fluids into me to compensate for the dehydration.

There was a problem, however. The nurse had trouble getting the IV started because of my dehydration. It actually took three people and many sticks before they could get into a vein. The surgeon walked in, saying, "Would you believe that this lady was out *running* this morning?" Under the influence of the numbing pre-op medication, I muttered: "See? No problem with running the day of surgery." That was the last thing I remembered.

The surgery went very well. I was wheeled from the operating room to the recovery room. As I was coming out of the anesthesia, I was already thinking about starting the exercises that the American Cancer Society's Reach to Recovery support group recommends. Because I was still pretty numb, I felt no pain and was raring to go. As I was trying to lift my arm, the surgeon walked in to check on me.

Looking perplexed, he asked, "What are you trying to do?"

"I've got to get started on my exercises!" I told him.

He patted me on the shoulder and said gently, "Oh, I think we can wait a couple of days."

"Oh, okay," I said and immediately fell back to sleep.

The next time I awoke, I *couldn't* move my arm. Each time I tried, there were sharp, stabbing pains. For a while, I tried to just gut through the increasing pain. When that didn't work, a fuzzy series of thoughts occurred to me: *This is only temporary. There's no point in suffering like this. I might as well be comfortable. That's what pain medication is for.* I succumbed to the siren call of the medication and slept.

The next morning, when I awoke, I began to wonder when I could try running again since I was feeling a lot better. When the doctor came by to check on me, I immediately popped the question.

"As soon as you feel like it," he said.

"Well," I replied, *"when* do you think I'll feel like it?"

He chuckled, "Oh, knowing you, probably in a couple of weeks." He beamed as though he thought that was just *wonderful* news.

"A couple of *weeks?*" I replied. I was expecting him to say a couple of days! I thought of all the conditioning I'd lose by not being able to run for two whole weeks.

After he left, I got out of bed. I started walking up and down the halls, pushing my IV stand, and preparing my body for a possible run the next day. That night, I awoke a number of times, the pain still intruding on my sleep. My body required more medication and more time. The second day after surgery, I was still a little weak and shaky on my feet. Disappointed, I thought, *Will I ever get back to running again?* It had been only two days, but it seemed like a month. On the third day, however, I felt great. "Today's the day!" I announced.

The poor nurses must have been in awe of this running-obsessed patient, and yet they were totally supportive. I asked for a wide elastic bandage to wrap around my chest. They brought me a twelve-inch-wide Ace wrap with which they then helped me swaddle myself so that nothing could move— not that there was much left that could bounce around, but it gave me a nice feeling of security. When the bandages were snug around me, I found that I could move with a lot less pain and could very carefully get into my running clothes. One of the nurses even offered to tie my shoe laces for me!

Triumphant, I walked out of the hospital and broke into a tentative, gingerly jog. It felt wonderful! Tears came again to my eyes. But this time, they were tears of joy!

CHAPTER ONE

MY RACE FOR LIFE

In this book is the story of how I decided to turn my life around through a combination of three major lifestyle changes: a whole-food, plant-based, low-fat vegan diet; extensive fitness training; and a "can do/must do/ will do whatever it takes" attitude. All three, I believe, have been vital in ensuring that more than forty years after my diagnosis, I have not had any recurrence of that potentially fatal cancer. I do know, however, that the risk of a recurrence still exists because cancer is so devious and can lie dormant for up to fifty years, waiting for another opportunity to strike.

With my new diet, I found that I was breaking state running records for my age group in the 5K, the 8K, the 10K, the 15K, the 25K, the 30K, the half marathon, and the marathon. I even boasted a surprise wheelchair-division first place.

How I "Won" a Wheelchair 5K Race

One Saturday afternoon, I was doing jumps on a trampoline when I landed on a pointed toe, fracturing the navicular, one of the bones in the mid-foot. The crack reverberated so loudly that there was no question that I had broken a bone. I was put on crutches.

I had a 5K race the next morning and could not cancel because I was the race director. By chance, we had a wheelchair division because we had one male entrant, Kim (who was a real pro at wheelchair racing and even had a special lightweight wheelchair just for races). As I watched him transfer to his racing wheelchair, I suddenly hated being left behind and got an idea. I asked Kim if he would mind if I tried doing the race in his regular wheelchair. He looked surprised but said, "Go for it!"

As soon as I fired the starting gun, I got into his other wheelchair and, of course, immediately got left in the dust. At the turnaround, because I was in last place, a police escort started following me very slowly all the way to the finish line. But as I was the only female wheelchair entrant, naturally, both Kim and I got first-place trophies.

This added to my collection of nearly a thousand first-place race trophies. I knew full well that it was the diet, not any innate ability, that was responsible. I was *not* doing all this to say, "Hey, look at me!" I was doing it to say, "Hey, look at how powerful a whole-food, plant-based, low-fat vegan diet is!"

In the next pages, I will talk about the importance of this diet in creating optimal health and providing the right nutrients for total fitness, strength, recovery, and resilience. I will offer my experience of being the first vegan and the first cancer patient to take part in one of the toughest races in the world, the Ironman triathlon, and finding life-altering challenges, great personal fulfillment, and companionship along the way. I will provide practical insights into how to train your body and create a positive attitude to face all of life's many challenges.

If all of this seems a little overwhelming, I don't blame you. I was overwhelmed at first too. I deeply believe that I am no more special or committed a person than anyone else. Like you, I have had moments of fear and doubt when I didn't know where to turn. But I also believe that we all have the resources in our minds and our bodies to help us overcome any challenge and leave us with a lasting sense of achievement.

As I near my century mark, I look forward to continuing my race for life with this very healthy lifestyle. I hope that my story inspires you—no matter how old or young you are or how physically challenged you may be—to stretch your capabilities and throw off the stereotypes attached with your age or your physical condition. If you are anything like me, you'll be amazed at what you can do. If you follow the plans and ideas in this book, you'll get results. Join me in this race for life!

Enter the Diet

If there is one cornerstone to my health, fitness, ability to prevent disease, and success in my treatment program, it would have to be nutrition. It's the food! After all, never did my fourteen years of daily running, my very positive mental attitude, and my belief that it could never happen to me, prevent my cancer from developing. The change in my diet happened thanks to both serendipity and curiosity. Just days after my diagnosis, I saw a tiny notice in a Honolulu newspaper that read:

> Breast cancer and diet study being conducted. Those who have or have had breast cancer are invited to join a study to determine the benefit of diet in the treatment of cancer. For further information, call Dr. John A. McDougall. 262- . . .

I couldn't believe my eyes. The timing was just perfect. If the notice had read, "to determine the benefit of cosmic radiation in the treatment of cancer," I would have been on the phone in a flash. I was totally desperate. The slightest promise of a cure—of salvation—is enough to get cancer patients like me to agree to being sent into orbit, if that's what it takes. I was no exception, and so I can easily understand why we grasp at quack cures. (You can read more about this later.) Moreover, I'd been told by both my surgeons and my oncologist that I could eat anything I wanted, that there was no way diet could have any influence on cancer. But here, all of a sudden, was hope!

I did not hesitate for a moment. I dialed the phone number listed and was shocked to find myself speaking to Dr. John McDougall. How often do you call a doctor's office and end up talking to the doctor themself? I nervously told him that I had just been diagnosed with breast cancer and that I had read his notice in the paper. He said: "Get your medical records and come to my office. I want to talk to you."

When I got there, newspaper clipping in hand (which, by the way, I still have and cherish), Dr. McDougall explained to me why he thought that diet is so important to cancer, that it can both initiate *and promote* cancer. I learned that breast cancer rates are low in countries with low-fat, low-animal-foods diets, while the opposite is true in countries such as the US, where diets are high in fat and animal foods.

So here was the answer to my question, "Why me?" I found out that a typical American gets more than 50 percent of their calories from low-quality carbohydrates and artery-clogging saturated fat, placing the Standard American Diet (SAD) among the fattiest in the world.[1] I also discovered that when women from countries with typically low-fat diets migrate to countries like ours and adopt higher-fat diets, the rates at which they get breast cancer soon approximate their destination countries' statistics. In other words, genetics does not seem to play a role in the development of cancer, nor, so it seemed, does age, considering the increase in incidence of breast cancer in all age groups and even in men. Even more important to me was the finding that when women in countries with low-fat diets get breast cancer, they live much longer.[2] This fact really got my attention. Here was hope. Here was a chance to extend my life.

Was there any question that I needed to change my diet? None! Absolutely none!

No Chemotherapy and Radiation

There was a little catch though. Dr. McDougall advised me not to undergo chemotherapy and radiation. I was quite surprised because I thought that in my case, considering the size of my tumor and the signs that it had spread, these treatments would be necessary. He explained that chemotherapy and radiation would permanently damage my immune system, whereas I was needing it the most. I needed my immune system to be in the best shape possible to stop the cancer now and prevent it from recurring in the future. I recall Dr. McDougall stating emphatically, "If you want to save your life, change your diet!"

I was confused. *Who do I believe? Which side should I go with?* When I asked about doing both, he told me: "Absolutely not, because if the diet works, they'll say it was the chemo and radiation. There can only be *one* variable in this research, and it's the diet." This was pretty scary now. There was one deciding factor, however, that helped me make my decision. Dr. McDougall pulled out the studies that supported what he was saying. The other doctors didn't.

I was now totally convinced. After two hours, I walked out of his office a confirmed vegan. I gave up all animal foods—including fish, dairy products, and eggs—and oils literally overnight and refused chemotherapy, radiation, and even the prescribed hormone-blockers.

When I got home, I excitedly told my husband what I'd learned, that it was my diet that had caused my breast cancer. I told him that Dr. McDougall was doing actual research on diet and cancer to prove this, that I was going to enroll in his study and be part of this research. I told him that this meant changing my diet to one with lots of starches such as potatoes and rice, vegetables, beans, and fruit. "What?" he said. "You can't eat any meat? No fish? No cheese? That's ridiculous! You've fallen into the hands of a very convincing quack. I gave you credit for more intelligence than that!"

The last bit really hurt especially because at the time, I was working on my PhD. I was so sure I had my husband's unconditional support. Back when we were given the bad news that it was cancer, I had fallen into his arms crying. He had hugged me tightly and started crying too. Having lost his first wife to cancer, he must have been hit hard. I thought he'd support me all through my fight against cancer, but now I saw that I was going to have to do this alone.

The Vegan Diet

Implementing Dr. McDougall's meal plan was simple: if something was of plant origin, I ate it; if it was of animal origin, I didn't. This diet is called "vegan," "strict vegetarian," or more recently, "whole-food plant-based," but you needn't worry about terminology. Right away, most people will have lots of questions: "Aren't chicken and fish good for you?" "Where would you get your protein?" "Where would you get your calcium?" "What's wrong with milk, yogurt, and cheese?" "What about iron?" "What's left to eat?" Lots! Don't worry. All of these questions will be answered in the course of this book.

Let me just say for now that the effects of my dietary change on my cancer were almost immediate. The horrible bone pain that had been plaguing me started subsiding within days. Then, in just twenty-one days, a new blood test showed that my sky-high liver enzymes had normalized and my cholesterol had dropped from a high of 236 mg/dL to 160 mg/dL. At the next test six months later, my cholesterol was a nice, low 128 mg/dL, and at the one after that, it was under 100! This practically eliminated my risk of having a heart attack, a scenario I hadn't ever even considered.

Indeed, back when Dr. McDougall saw my initial reading of 236 mg/dL, he told me that I was at as great a risk of dying of a heart attack as of the cancer! Another great health shocker, considering that as a marathoner, I had thought I was immune to heart disease. (This was just before Jim Fixx, one of the most famous of all runners and author of *The Complete Book of Running*, died of a heart attack at age fifty-two in 1984.)

I was shocked that my cholesterol could be so high; after all, I was a heavy exerciser and had long given up red meat. What I didn't know then was that chicken and fish have just as much cholesterol as do beef and pork—that muscle is muscle, whether it moves a hoof, a wing, or a fin. I had not done my body any favors by switching the source of cholesterol. I also saw that exercise in general, even when it's marathon running, sure does not lower cholesterol levels.

It's not surprising that people think they're eating more healthily by choosing chicken and fish instead of beef and pork. The meat industries omit cholesterol levels altogether, thus the cholesterol in chicken and fish remains hidden. Here, for instance, is an advertisement for beef that ran nationally in a popular magazine:

Cholesterol: perception vs. reality. This should make headlines: lean, trimmed beef has no more cholesterol than chicken—without the skin.

Similarly, a fast-food chain advertised: "Our mouth-watering ribs are as low in cholesterol as chicken and fish."

The beef and pork industries must be hoping that their verbal manipulation gets past the public's awareness that the cholesterol content must be the same in all animal meat—about 25 milligrams per ounce of muscle, to be precise, regardless of the type of animal. (After all, it's animal muscle that you're eating whether you're eating steak, a hamburger, ribs, a roast, or a drumstick.) In this case, even "low-cholesterol" means "high-cholesterol."

When I saw all the benefits from my diet change and understood the underlying science, I kept trying to convince my husband that this new diet could help him too. He had high blood pressure as well as other problems for which he was taking prescribed drugs. He responded with, "How could a breast-cancer diet be good for all these other diseases?" He did ask his doctor if I could be right, and the doctor told him what he wanted to hear—that diet had nothing to do with his high blood pressure and that he'd be on medication for the rest of his life. What I didn't know at the time was that my "breast-cancer diet" would also be the "heart-disease diet," the "stroke diet," the "diabetes diet," the "weight-loss diet," and, as it turned out, my "Ironman diet." We now know that the SAD diet is the root cause of almost every one of the chronic, degenerative diseases we have in this country.[3]

Dismissed by both my husband and my oncologist, who insisted that diet couldn't have caused my breast cancer, I was nevertheless grateful for the support and guidance that I got from Dr. McDougall and his wife Mary. I continued to research and learn more about all of the many benefits of a whole-food, plant-based, low-fat vegan diet. This diet is valuable not just to human health but also to all those poor animals some call "food" and to the environment, which is ravaged by animal husbandry.

Enter Exercise

Running had become a daily fixture in my life since 1968, thanks to a particular man and a particular book. I was in a newsstand looking for something to read before boarding a long flight when I happened to see the word "aerobics" for the first time, which, as it turned out, Dr. Kenneth Cooper had just coined following his research on the benefits of exercise—such as running, cycling, swimming, and cross-country skiing—that involves all the major muscle groups. I thumbed through Dr. Cooper's *Aerobics*, became curious about what he'd found, and bought the book, which I finished on that plane ride.

The next morning, I dug out my old tennis shoes from the back of the closet, put them on along with a pair of cuffed Bermuda shorts and an old t-shirt, and went out for my first run. I ran down to the end of my street and back. When I got back, I got into my car and, using the odometer, found out that I'd run a whole mile. I was hooked! I started running in the early morning every day before going to work; soon, I was feeling stronger and more energetic, and I even enjoyed my runs. I could eat more and not worry about gaining extra weight, something I had been wary of before. I did have a minor concern about what people would think when they saw me running. Remember that this was back in 1968, several years before the "running boom" started in 1972, when anyone who was seen running on streets was assumed to be trying to catch a bus or running from the police after having committed a crime. It was that rare a scene back then.

After reading the ground-breaking book *Aerobics*, I got interested in all forms of exercise and its many benefits, which I learned include the delivery of oxygen and nutrients to all parts of the body, especially the brain. The muscle-pumping action of exercise also decreases the risk of potentially fatal blood clots.

It has been said that exercise is the body's second heart. It's also the only way to keep your lymph, which stagnates when you are sitting, circulating. The contraction of muscles moves the lymph fluid around. (With three times the volume of blood but no pump like the heart, lymph fluid is the body's main detoxification system that keeps the blood clean, kind of like a garbage disposal.)

In addition, exercise encourages the production of nitric oxide, a molecule produced by the epithelial lining of the arteries that allows them to relax, lowers blood pressure, and increases blood flow. During my research, I also learned that resistance (load-bearing) exercise or lifting weights is the way to increase muscle mass, increase bone density, and fight off sarcopenia, the progressive and generalized loss of muscle in aging. There are more benefits that I learned about as I earned my qualification as a personal fitness trainer, but more on this later.

It is worth reemphasizing that I got into regular exercising only as an adult. Other than running around as most children do, I was never particularly athletic when I was younger, although I did swim. I grew up in Lanikai, Hawaii, across the street from the beach, so this was only natural. I kept up my swimming and at one point was even the only girl on my high-school swim team, which was kind of fun.

My First Race
Back in 1970, when I was the chief of an all-male military office, one of the sergeants who worked for me handed me a flyer announcing a road race. He knew I was a regular runner and said I ought to do it. Thinking that it might be fun, I signed up.

As I showed up on race day and looked around, I could see nothing but fit-looking, young men. I was the only female. I began to have second thoughts. *What am I doing here? What if I come in last? What if I can't even finish?* This didn't seem like such a good idea now. I was afraid of embarrassing myself and even all of womankind. I was ready to quietly slink away, but it was too late. The starting gun went off, and I was nearly trampled. To avoid getting run over, I ran all out and almost died at the half-mile mark. My chest and lungs were screaming in pain, my legs turned to lead, and I felt as if I was dying. I had no choice but to slow down to nearly a walk. Slowly, I recovered enough to get back up to a halfway-decent pace. When, at long last, I saw the finish line, I put on a final sprint. After crossing the finish line, I looked around to see that I wasn't even last. Having completed my first race, I happily collected my very first trophy, a gold medal.

How to Make "Hard" Seem "Easy"

I would not forget the excruciating pains I had felt during my first race and started training to increase my speed and endurance. My next race was a four-miler, and my experience running it was essentially a repeat of my first. With no other women in competition yet again, I was rewarded with my second first-place trophy. Having survived twice now, I entered a ten-kilometer (6.2-mile) race.

I noticed that the same sequence occurred no matter what the distance of the race and that a race could be divided into a beginning, a middle, and an end. The beginning started great but ended when all those horrible pains in my chest and legs creeped in. The middle began as I slowed my pace and the pains subsided. The end began when I saw the finish line. I'd speed up and try to just hang on until I crossed it. In every race, this sequence played out the same—except in a longer race, the middle began later and lasted longer.

It would be another four years before I attempted a half-marathon. And as you might be able to guess, I went through the exact same sequence. By then, I'd amassed enough experience to know that regardless of distance, the ending was the same: I would cross the finish line with the little that I had left. I did not realize then that this is the way it's supposed to be—you give it your all!

The leap from a half-marathon to a full marathon was a greater psychological battle, and I took the plunge only when I realized that three of the military guys working for me had each completed a marathon with much less training (though admittedly, they were ten to twenty years younger than I was). I thought that if they could do it, so could I. I decided to break through both barriers—sex and age. Fueled by this new determination, I kept extending my long runs, gaining much confidence along the way.

As I crossed the finish line at the end of my first marathon, I realized that I'd once again gone through the sequence of beginning, middle, and end, with nothing left at the end.

Four years later, I began to train for my first ultra-marathon (defined as any race with a distance longer than the standard marathon distance of 26.2 miles). Once my goal became an ultra, the marathon seemed almost easy by comparison. It was a most exciting discovery—that when I set a higher goal, anything less than that would be doable, even easy.

Setting a New Path

Have you ever noticed the amount of activity in a colony of ants? Have you observed how purposeful the ants seem to be? Each member of the group seems to know where to go, what to do, and when to do it. These ants' entire lives are wrapped up in accomplishing genetically programmed goals.

Now look at us humans. Some people seem to know what to do, how to do it, and when to do it. I never felt that fortunate. It seemed as though I was always looking at a whole bunch of options, finding myself wanting more than one, then looking back at the choices I'd made and wishing I'd done something else.

With my diagnosis, all of that got swept away. On my daily runs high up on Pearl Ridge on Oahu where I lived, looking down, I saw, as if for the first time, the crystalline blue of the waters of Pearl Harbor and the lush green of the palm trees. Suddenly, just being alive was the essence of my life; everything else was secondary. Then came a new and exhilarating sense of almost reckless abandon and excitement for the opportunities that were to come.

I looked back at my life and saw the times when I'd been one of those ants, just following the trail marked by the ant in front. I'd not dared to strike out on a trail of my own making. Cancer did for me what I had been unable to do on my own. It plucked me from the trail of conventionality and dropped me in another place, one that seemed unique. Yes, other people had been diagnosed with cancer, but each had had their own situation. For quite a while after the diagnosis, it appeared that I was not going to die immediately. I felt freed to think in new ways about the rest of my life.

Running around the World

It was one of the early days after my diagnosis. I was sitting in the hospital waiting room, waiting for my second chest x-ray after the first one had shown a very suspicious lesion in my lung. Fearing the worst, I felt tears welling up. Then I looked at the man sitting across from me. It occurred to me that maybe he was facing an even worse diagnosis. I asked him if he was here for a chest x-ray too. He said that he was with the consulate in China and was here for his routine annual exam. My ears perked up at the word "China." I told him that I'd always dreamed of running on the Great Wall but that now it was too late—I'd gotten breast cancer. He reached into his vest pocket and pulled out his card. He said: "You will do it! Call me when you get to China."

Encouraged, I started visualizing myself actually running along that magnificent ancient creation. The next year, I started planning a trip to China. I created and realized a fantastic dream. In 1983, one year after my diagnosis, I ran the Great Wall of China—well, not its entire length. So much of it is in a state of disrepair; plus, it's over 1,300 miles. Nonetheless, I ran enough of it to get to feel like I had accomplished something close to impossibility, considering my old frame of reference.

Running along that majestic wall was a joy in itself, but the real thrill for me came from seeing the surprised looks on all the locals' faces. Back in 1983, when China had just started opening its borders to tourists, most Chinese people had never seen a tall, fair Western woman, much less one in a running singlet and shorts; they must have thought I was crazy. After all, why would anyone want to run when they didn't have to?

Waves of dropped-jawed Chinese people parted and gawked in awe as I threaded my way through. They pointed at me, smiles playing around their eyes. Then their lips widened, and their whole faces beamed. One elderly gentleman playfully ran alongside me, laughing uproariously. He was saying something in Chinese, and I was telling him that I'd just been diagnosed with cancer, but look, here I was! Despite my speaking in English and he in Chinese, we communicated soul to soul perfectly, and I know that for a few precious moments, we enriched each other's lives.

That was the beginning of my running all around the world, literally—which, as a matter of fact, I have done twice now. The first time, I went by air, the second by ship. Running is an exciting way to see new countries and meet people of different cultures who share a love of the sport.

After returning from China, I decided to backpack across Haleakala, the 10,023-foot-high volcano on the island of Maui known as the "House of the Sun." As I scampered down the shale of the inside of the crater of the extinct volcano, I was hoping all the while that the volcanologists were right in their assessment, that Haleakala really was extinct. I peered down seemingly bottomless crevasses, saw two spectacular sunrises, and ran up the far side of the crater in a quarter of the time usually allotted for people to climb out.

I felt the same as I had in China—that this was really living—and I wondered why I had waited so long to start! At the time, I had not yet even conceived of running the 36.6-mile Run to the Sun from Kahului to the top of Haleakala, from sea level to 10,023-foot altitude. The following year, I did it, completing it in seven hours and forty-seven minutes and winning an age-group first place.

I continued to set new challenges for myself as I reaped the benefits of my new diet—increased strength and resilience and fast recovery. In 1986, the fourth year after my diagnosis, I ran fifty-one races and placed in almost every one of them: thirty-three first places, nine second places, and three thirds; the remaining six races were "fun runs" with no times or awards. The races ranged from one-mile all-out sprints to Ironman triathlons; I managed to establish numerous course, state, and international age-group records in running, biking, and swimming, in triathlons and even a pentathlon at the age of sixty-four.

In 1987, the fifth year after my cancer diagnosis, I did fifty-two races, again ranging in distances from the mile to the Ironman triathlon, with even more first-place awards. In 1988, I changed my focus a little and ran the Moscow Marathon, plus races in St. Petersburg and Sochi, then still more races in Kyiv and Kharkov in Ukraine. This was before the Berlin Wall came down, when there were still animosities between the

Communist countries and the West, and well before the unbelievably tragic attack on Ukraine in 2022. As our interpreters told the Russians and Ukrainians we met about me, this fifty-three-year-old cancer patient who did Ironman triathlons, they had looks of amazement on their faces that I will never forget. They wanted to know everything about my diet and training schedule, about how I got myself to do all of these things. I delighted in the opportunity to talk about the importance of diet, exercise, and an overall healthy lifestyle.

The Moscow Marathon

The Moscow Marathon was one of the more exotic marathons that I've entered and certainly one of my most memorable. Since I wanted to take the "aloha" spirit to the USSR, I carried as part of my baggage five thousand Hawaiian orchids, to be distributed to the spectators along the course. It was wonderful to behold the expressions of surprise and delight on the faces of the Russian people. The experience was even more unique thanks to the course marshals, who were all soldiers from the Russian army and who stood shoulder to shoulder at attention, rigid and stone-faced, along the entire 26.2-mile route. While handing them orchids, I wanted to tell them that I'd come all the way from Hawaii to run in their marathon. They'd just look at me, totally puzzled, as I repeated, "Hawaii." They did not understand the word because there is no *h* sound in their language. When my interpreter told me that the Russian pronunciation for "Hawaii" was *Ga-vai* and I finally pronounced it right, they understood, nodding their heads, with eyes dancing and big smiles on their faces. I spent so much time talking to foreign runners during that marathon that I had a terribly slow time, a PW (personal worst). But do you think that mattered?

After the marathon, running through the streets of Moscow, I found that the Russians were intensely curious about Americans. They were extremely friendly and usually knew enough English to carry on a limited conversation. Being able to communicate with hundreds of people from immensely different backgrounds was hugely rewarding for me.

In 1989, I spent three weeks in Thailand and Nepal, entering every race I could find. It was a similar experience there too. There were many opportunities for me to mix with the local people, share my experiences,

13

and tell my story. People in those places, especially in Kathmandu, Nepal, could not understand why anyone would exert so much effort when it wasn't really necessary for survival. The concept of exercise was completely foreign to them, many of whom engaged in heavy labor all day long, barely eking out a living.

Nepal as a nation was so poverty-stricken that it seemed almost criminal to waste any of the body's energy. Food there was such a limited commodity and life there was so hard that the Nepalese didn't even have a choice in what to eat. People already had an extremely low-fat diet; they "exercised" the whole day and half the night—and seven days a week at that.

I also saw that the levels of stress people there were under were extremely high. I mentally compared the stressors that affected them with those that affected us Americans back home (deadlines, traffic congestion, noise pollution, etc.). These people worked long, hard days with no "coffee breaks" and rarely any days off. Even with all the heavy labor, some were not making a subsistence-level living. Many could hardly feed their children; I couldn't imagine a greater stressor. I had previously wondered if stress had played a role in my getting breast cancer, but when I saw real stress, I realized that the types of stress I was experiencing in my life were rather minor.

Ironically, I thought, the Nepalese were on average very healthy; they lived and remained active to ripe old ages. For them, obesity didn't exist; neither did heart disease, most forms of cancer, ulcers, diabetes, osteoporosis, high blood pressure, arthritis, or dementia. Out the door went the theories that stress causes ulcers and high blood pressure, that insufficient consumption of dairy products causes osteoporosis, and that osteoarthritis is attributable to "wear and tear" (see later chapters for more on these subjects). As a result of the very positive changes in the way I felt and looked, I came to believe that diet plays by far the most important role in ensuring survival, health, and athletic capability at any age. I believe that my new diet was mostly responsible for shooting me into the international sports arena.

One of the Ten Fittest Women

In May 1998, *Living Fit* magazine sponsored a contest to seek the "ten fittest women of 1999." When a friend suggested that I enter, I thought I wouldn't stand a chance because at sixty-four, I was so much older than those typically seen in fitness magazines. But because of my long-term commitment to daily exercise, I felt like here was an opportunity to prove that age does not necessarily define fitness. Needless to say, I was pretty excited when I was notified, first by phone and then by an official express-delivery letter, that I was one of the ten chosen.

At last, as a *mature* woman (by the way, I no longer consider sixty-four "old"), I felt as though I'd come into my own. No longer did I consider myself an ancient relic to be put on the shelf or in a rocking chair; I was one to be reckoned with in the sports world. Who'd have thought that anyone could go from bearer of a devastating metastatic-cancer diagnosis to world-champion Ironman triathlete and one of the fittest women in the world?

But what is the Ironman triathlon? And how did I get involved in it?

Chapter Two

Enter the Ironman

Watching the Ironman on TV

In 1982, after my first mastectomy, I was on medical leave and had some time to watch television. While channel surfing, I happened to come across the *ABC Wide World of Sports'* coverage of the Ironman World Championship Triathlon, an event that consisted of an open-ocean swim of 2.4 miles, a bike race of 112 miles, and finally a full marathon, which is 26.2 miles. I watched, intrigued, as amazing events like this unfolded, my eyes glued to the screen. I could hardly believe what I was seeing. Having run several marathons, I knew how I felt at the end of one; in that instant, it seemed impossible for me to even consider doing a marathon *after* having had to swim and bike first.

What I saw next was one of the most famous incidents in sports history. Julie Moss, in first place and approaching the finish line, collapsed from total exhaustion. She struggled to get up, collapsing again. As she tried once more to get up, the crowd of spectators shouted encouraging words, "Get up, Julie, get up!" but she could not as her body was starting to shut down. She started crawling, got to within what seemed like just inches from the finish line, then finally crossed it, but in the meantime, Kathleen McCartney, having no idea of the drama that was playing out, had crossed the line first.

Watching Julie Moss's heroic effort made me realize I had a similar crisis in my own life. I was a marathoner one day, a cancer patient the next! I decided right then that I was going to do the Ironman triathlon.

Watching the Ironman in Person

While on medical leave to recover from my reconstruction surgery, I treated myself to visiting my dad, who happened to live in Kona, on the Big Island.

My visit was timed, not coincidentally, with the running of the 1983 Kona Ironman Triathlon. Now that I got to see an Ironman in person, I was even more amazed by this grueling event than when I had seen it on TV. Standing on the sidelines, I watched, awestruck, as competitors completed the 2.4-mile swim, dashed out of the water and climbed onto their bikes for the 112-mile bike race, then dropped their bikes to start the 26.2-mile marathon. My brain had trouble taking it all in.

One side of my brain went: "This is humanly impossible! No one can do this much! It can't be done!"

"Yes, it can!" replied the other side.

"No, it can't! It's impossible."

"No, it isn't. Look, if they can do it, maybe . . . !"

"No, no, nope, no way!"

This went on for hours as I saw so many of the finishers struggle to make it to the finish line within the cut-off time of seventeen hours. I recalled again how I often felt upon crossing a marathon finish line—totally spent, exhausted, with absolutely nothing left! How could these people run a full marathon after a swim that took the average competitor from one to over two hours *and* a bike ride that took six to eight hours, all under extreme heat? Since the start was at 7 a.m., the final hurdle, the marathon, had to be completed by midnight to escape disqualification. The reality that many of the competitors had been going full-bore for close to those seventeen hours hit me with an intensity I couldn't believe.

As I continued to watch, an idea formed in my head, but a different idea this time. "Maybe I *could* do that." Again, the two voices battled it out inside my head.

"No, I couldn't possibly."

"Well, maybe I can."

"Forget it, that's crazy."

"Maybe if I train hard enough."

"No way, it's impossible! Besides, you're way too old." (Age forty-seven seemed absolutely ancient to me at the time.)

"Well, maybe I could just try it. . . ."

"My God, lady, even if you weren't too old, you're forgetting you're now a cancer patient!"

And thus, this internal dialogue ended . . . but then, it would begin again. An image of me crossing that finish line was constantly in my mind. During my daily runs, I would picture that scene in Kona, Hawaii: the large finish-line clock, the tropical flowers surrounding the finish area, and the cheering crowds.

Yet, I still wasn't sure. I told myself that there had to be a limit to what I was physically able to do, and I did not want to set myself up for probable failure by reaching for something that was totally out of reach. I thought again about Julie Moss and her heroic effort to cross that finish line. But surely, for a middle-aged cancer patient, this quest seemed totally ridiculous. My self-doubt was validated by the fact that at that time, no woman that old had ever completed the Ironman. Remember: we're talking about a race that has a cut-off time of seventeen hours, running from 7 a.m. until midnight; lots of competitors don't make it! I told myself that it would be absolute lunacy for me, someone handicapped by both age and cancer, to even contemplate such a feat.

Yet, my mind would continue to wander. Images of my getting stronger kept coming up, and from time to time, the thought of doing the Ironman would reappear. I started biking daily and right away began to push the limits in terms of both the distance and the intensity of my rides. I signed up for a master's (adult) swim class, not really knowing if I could do it. I had to keep drumming up that positive attitude that everybody keeps referencing.

With all of this new activity came the determination to prove to the world how powerful my diet was. My vision became clear: "A vegan cancer patient completed the Ironman triathlon." During my training, I kept thinking about those contrasting concepts—"vegan," "cancer," and "Ironman"—and I was intrigued. Wouldn't I then prove to myself and the world that I really was a survivor, that I had beaten the disease with my vegan diet that so many thought was deficient in protein and calcium? What if I took that damning diagnosis of cancer and turned it into the challenge of a lifetime, becoming an "Ironman" in the process? What if extreme super-fitness could help fight cancer? What if getting my body to become the fittest it had ever been in my whole life was the best offense against the cancer cells that surely remained in my body? It was an exciting goal, something to wrap my life around, something worthy of a major commitment, for I knew it would take up a large part of my life.

I knew I was falling in love with the Ironman. I started getting more serious about all three of the sports involved and even added weight lifting. I subscribed to all the magazines, poring over them cover to cover. I looked for anything written about the triathlon that I could find, not that there was much in those early days of the event. I started examining the training schedule of every athlete I ran into. My obsession was total.

Then I noticed the physical and mental changes. My muscles became more defined, and it seemed new ones kept popping up all over. One morning, as a friend, Bonnie K., and I were walking to a race start line, she paused and looked down at me in mock disgust, shaking her head, "You and your 'thirty-year-old' legs!"

I slept like a rock and awakened sometimes after only five or six hours of sleep, raring to go for my morning run, which ended only when I'd run out of time. I ate like a horse and never gained a pound; in fact, I had to eat a lot to keep myself from losing weight. I felt strong and confident, and as if for the first time, I was really enjoying life. I had found a challenge that was totally engrossing. I could even forget about the cancer for short periods of time, and more importantly, I felt that I was onto something in dealing with it.

What if there really never would be a cure? What if strengthening the body's immune system was the only way to deal with cancer? I remembered that when I'd asked my oncologist how to help my body fight the cancer, he had replied while shaking his head, "Nobody knows."

I developed a theory revolving around diet and exercise that took both to an extreme, although I now know that it doesn't have to be as extreme as I'd originally thought. I found it ironic that diet-oriented physicians disagreed with my approach to exercise and exercise-oriented physicians disagreed with my dietary approach. Back then, nobody, as far as I knew, had ever put the two together. It was scary wading into uncharted waters, but after all, I felt that I had little to lose and so much to gain.

The body craves and *needs* movement. When given enough time to adapt, it can accomplish prodigious feats. This was true for even my nearly fifty-year-old body that, years earlier, I'd thought was already old! I was feeling younger, and I certainly did not fit the stereotypes of how an older woman like me should look and act. There are truly no limits, I concluded—only those we set in our own minds.

My First Ironman

My philosophy worked: I graduated from my first triathlon, the Tinman (approximately a quarter-Ironman), in 1982, then I moved on to a half-Ironman, then to a full one. Training for my first Tinman, I knew so little about cycling that I thought as long as I could cover the distance just once, that was good enough. It was only after that first Tinman that I knew better. It being the first time I had to go all out for the full 25 miles on the bicycle, I was shocked to discover that when I got off the bike, my legs were like rubber. I was staggering and could hardly walk, much less be ready to start the 10K run. I did eventually manage to get through it with the realization that I needed more training on the bike and that when racing on the bike, I had to go through the exact same sequence as when running a race: the beginning, with the accompanying chest and leg pains; the middle, when I would back off enough to withstand the pain; and the end, when the finish line was in sight. That was a major discovery for me and, I suspect, most of those who were just venturing into the world of triathlons in those early days, when there were no experts to turn to and no texts to consult.

Then there was the matter of increasing distances. The Tinman Triathlon's swim segment was a half-mile, the bike leg was 25 miles, and the run was a 10K (6.2 miles). The first half-Ironman–distance triathlon in Hawaii was the Windward Triathlon in 1983. While the 1.2-mile swim didn't seem too bad, the 56-mile bike leg had me worried as I recalled my first Tinman's bike-leg finish. Then, when I had somehow conquered the 56-miler, looking at the 112-mile bike leg of the Ironman, I was totally awed by that distance and 56 miles again became a piece of cake by comparison. The process of increasing my running distance was the same, although significantly more challenging because of the fatigue factor.

Shortly after winning gold in one of the Tinman triathlons, I was interviewed by a reporter from a local weekly magazine called *Midweek*. I was already excited when my picture appeared on the next issue's cover with the headline "A Grandmother Fights Cancer and Trains for the Ironman." Little did I know that there would be a deeper meaning to that headline. Just seven weeks before my first Ironman, a totally unexpected challenge presented itself when I found myself in a hospital bed, having been hit by a truck. I'll talk about that later in my chapter on accidents.

Getting to Meet Dr. Cooper

In 1989, I found out, with much excitement, that Dr. Cooper was coming to Honolulu to give a talk on aerobics. I, of course, attended. After his talk, I went backstage, introduced myself, and handed him a copy of the first draft of this book. I told him how his book had been responsible for the start of my lifelong passion for running, twenty years before, and how I would love to have his endorsement.

Two weeks later, I received a call from Dr. Cooper, who said that he could hardly believe what he'd just read, that a cancer patient with such a "weird" diet could do Ironman triathlons. He invited me to the now-world-famous Cooper Aerobics Research Center in Dallas, Texas, because he wanted to "run every test in the book" on me to see how I could do what I was doing. Then he said he would give me the chance to set a new women's *world* fitness record for my age group. He chuckled, "I suspect you will do it." I was to get on a treadmill that started out slowly and increased in both speed and incline, following a standard Balke protocol. When I reached exhaustion—sooner or later, since the machine would always win—my time was noted and compared to those of others in my age group.

This was a fantastic opportunity for me to demonstrate the importance of both diet and exercise to fitness. I first broke the record for the 55–59 age group in 1990, then broke my own record the following year, and then went back when I turned sixty and broke that record as well. It almost made me anxious to get older (well, not really, but at least there are some rewards).

Extra! Extra! Read All about It!

After the publicity I got in *Midweek*, an amazing series of events ensued. I got a call from a Continental Airlines agent, Dennis, with an offer of sponsorship. It was the dream of all the top triathletes to get sponsored, and here I was, just one of the hundreds doing the Ironman, receiving an offer. I was amazed. Of course, I asked what this would involve. Dennis said that they'd enter me in the New Zealand Triathlon in March. They'd supply me with sportswear with CONTINENTAL AIRLINES printed on it, which I'd wear while competing. They'd fly me there and cover all my expenses. This would occur just six months after I had done the Kona Ironman. I thought about the common belief that the Ironman was so grueling that it would take a whole *year* to fully recover after an event. However, I knew that with my new diet, my recovery would be a lot faster. I could not pass up this fantastic offer!

It turned out that I was right, because all went well with the competition, and I got first place in my age group. In addition to my own excitement, I could feel the excitement of others, as attested to by my picture on the front page of the *New Zealand Herald* the next day. The headline across the top read, "Ruth, A Woman of Iron!"

When I laid that issue of the *New Zealand Herald* with me on the front page on Dennis's desk once I was back from New Zealand, he looked down at it, looked up at me, smiled, and said, "Don't they have an Ironman in Japan coming up in August?" When I realized that it was only five months away, I thought, *There is no way I could do a third Ironman in less than a year. Doesn't Dennis realize that I've already done two Ironman triathlons in less than six months?*

My next thought was a devious one. *What if I can't finish? What are they going to do, fire me?* So, I said, "Yes, I'll do it!" I fully expected to have to lower my goals as far as my performance was concerned; to my surprise, I did very well and again placed first in my age group. This time, the headline in the Japanese newspaper *Asahi Shimbun* read, "American Woman, 54, Conquers Cancer, Conquers Ironman."

Another Example of Faster Recovery

The morning after completing the Japan Ironman, I was ready to go see the sights. One attraction, the famous Nara Park with its many deer, was only twenty-two miles—a short bus ride—away. I asked around to see if the other American triathletes would like to go with me to Nara Park.

Invariably, each one's response was along the lines of: "Are you kidding? I'm too sore." So I decided to go alone. As I got on the bus, I saw that I was the only *haole* (Hawaiian for "foreigner").

During the bus ride, I was enjoying the scenery when I noticed a Japanese newspaper rolled up in the back pocket of the seat in front of me. It was all in Japanese, which I couldn't read, but with an inkling that there might be some photos of the Ironman the day before, I opened it up and there was *me* at the finish line! I reflexively gasped, "Oh my God, it's me—that's me!" Showing it to the gentleman sitting across the aisle (who turned out to be a professor of English at the University of Kyoto), I gestured, pointing to myself and then to the photo. He reached for the paper, took a minute to read it, and smiled. He stood up and read the article to all the passengers, who gave a great round of applause!

I marveled at the incredible sequence of events that had brought me to this moment. First, my diet was allowing me to recover quickly enough to play tourist the day after completing an Ironman triathlon. Then I got on a bus and just happened to pick the seat with that newspaper, and sitting in the seat across from me was a Japanese professor who just happened to teach English. Surely, I must be dreaming. *This can't be happening*, I thought, but happening it was! I couldn't have written a better movie script. It was surreal!

Two Months Later, Another Ironman

Coming up in October was a new Kona Ironman, which I'd entered since I'd qualified in the one the year before. I wasn't sure that I could do another one, as this would be my fourth Ironman in just under a year (the previous Kona Ironman had been in late October and the one coming up was in early October). I decided that I'd test my limits and demolish the idea that it took a full year to recover from an Ironman. As long as I gave my body the right fuel and adequate rest time, my recovery would be fast. People, especially my coaches, were always telling me that I was racing too much, but maybe I could keep racing as frequently as I wanted. I had not yet realized then just how incredibly fast my recovery was becoming thanks to my new diet. Since both the New Zealand Ironman and the Japan Ironman had gone so well, I decided to take on the Kona Ironman as well.

So, on October 11, 1986, as I sat at Honolulu International Airport, awaiting my flight to Kailua-Kona for my fifth Ironman triathlon in a year, I marveled that I was even there. I recounted my journey in the past year: Just seven months before, I was on my way to enter an Ironman in New Zealand. With that age-group first place, I felt as though I was on top of the athletic world. That was in March, only five months after I'd done the 1985 Kona Ironman. Then there was the Japan Ironman, which I'd done just two months before. And now, I was off to yet another Ironman. I wasn't at all sure that I could meet the challenge.

After I crossed the finish line of the Kona Ironman a second time, my heart was racing. I realized then that I had really done it! I had accomplished a feat that, just a year ago, in the world of triathletes, had been deemed impossible. Who'd have thought that a now-fifty-one-year-old cancer patient could complete four Ironman triathlons in less than a year—and a vegan cancer patient at that! All of the mental and physical limits I'd been setting for myself had just been broken. Since then, my races have only continued to increase in number year after year and I have only continued to become stronger and faster, now with nearly a thousand trophies and medals to show for it.

In later chapters, I will cover training for the three events of the Ironman—swimming, biking, and running—although you don't have to run out and do an Ironman to reap the benefits of exercise. Just know that I believe that you can do it if you really want to. Even if you don't want to run, bike, or swim, there are other exercises that are similarly beneficial. Try jumping rope, climbing stairs, lifting weights, and even dancing! It all helps.

CHAPTER THREE

GETTING INFORMED

Triathletes are among the most sociable people I have ever met. I recall that during the early days, any of the questions I posed to them concerning any of the three sports was invariably answered totally, completely, and enthusiastically. The sharing of information seemed to be done so joyfully, and I found that as I learned the tricks of the trade, I, too, felt compelled to share what I knew with others, to the extent that I became a coach for ten years.

First, I would respond to people who asked for help. Next, I started voluntarily sharing information—as in, "Guess what I just found out!" Now, I share my knowledge in the form of interviews, seminars, radio talk shows, books, and videos, with the hope of reaching people who never dreamed of wanting to know all about the joys of exercise, particularly running, swimming, and cycling.

As I witnessed and participated in the sharing of information, experience, and advice, I noticed that unfortunately, there was, from time to time, misinformation that was widely passed on. Indeed, I even fell victim to some of these "fads," and it took me a long time to sort fact from fancy. It's a process that is far from ended, by the way, as the sport continuously progresses, as new equipment, techniques, and strategies are developed and become available to the people training and competing.

How to Keep Elephants Out of Your Backyard

Consider this method for keeping elephants out of your backyard. All you have to do is, at exactly six o'clock every evening, sprinkle some pure salt over your back gate.

"But," says your friend, "you don't have any elephants in your backyard!"

"See? It works!"

Keeping the elephants out is an analogy for superstitious behavior that sustains itself because it never fails to work. This kind of rationale goes on all around you. See if you can spot some real-life examples of elephant repellents.

In the early days following my cancer diagnosis, a number of people would approach me with possible "cures," some of which were so far out that I didn't even consider them. I did wonder, however, why so many others did. There were even glowing testimonies about the success rates of these cures, but they were invariably proved useless when the patients died anyway.

How "Snake-Oil" Cures Work

Take any large group of patients with a terminal disease and you'll find that for most, regardless of how serious the disease is, its course is never a straight line from diagnosis to inexorable death. There are good days and there are bad days. This is known as the "natural variability of disease."[1] At any given point, you'd catch some patients during their bad days—at the bottom and starting back up. If you were to give all of the patients a dose of snake oil or some such preparation, the patients just coming out of their bad days would assume that the snake oil made them better. We all have a tendency to want to create cause-and-effect links even when there may be none. When this happens, you've got a group of believers!

Those who are in between the good days and bad days or who are at the top then just need to be told that they need to keep on taking their doses of snake oil, that it takes time for the snake oil to work. You probably won't hear from most of these patients again anyway, so your reputation is safe. As for those who died, it is "obvious" that they hadn't started their snake-oil treatment soon enough.

If a self-proclaimed "expert" were to look deeply into your eyes and give you a diagnosis of "toxins in your lymphatics," and if you were to then spend a lot of money on the recommended snake-oil remedy to rid your body of these "toxins," it would be rude of your body not to feel better. Then, when you return for a follow-up visit a week later, this same "expert" would look deeply into your eyes again and pronounce you cured! The placebo effect is extremely powerful.

The Knowledge Boxes

A useful way to look at the total of all knowledge in the universe as it relates to us is as four boxes. In the first box is all that we know we know. In the second box is all that we don't know and that we *know* we don't know. In the third box is all that we know but don't *know* we know. And finally, in the fourth box is all that we don't know we don't know. Most of us are pretty comfortable with operating in the first and second boxes. Much of what we do day to day, we do automatically because we know what we know. We know that we know how to get to work, for example. We know that we don't know how to get to a street we've never heard of. We know we need a map in that case. Knowing what we don't know usually keeps us from getting in over our heads and getting in trouble.

All the information in the third box is what limits us. We don't know what we are really capable of because we never think to test it and, preferably, use it. Examples include athletic capability, leadership ability, or entrepreneurial skill that is untapped because it seems too scary to try.

The fourth box, however—what we don't know we don't know—holds the most potential. That's where the Great Beyond lies, where even our unconscious has never been able to reach to grasp knowledge. We can tap into the fourth box only when we open ourselves up to others more knowledgeable than we are. We can then be taken to realms that perhaps we didn't even know existed. These realms are different for each one of us. I was introduced to a whole new realm of dietary knowledge thanks to Dr. John McDougall.

Imagine a group of people who have always lived in a dense forest, never even suspecting that there are places beyond the forest, such as deserts, mountains, oceans, and space. These forest-dwellers may never know what they don't know. Or take fish for example. They know a lot about water but they don't know that they know all of this. This is why our mental capacities hold so much potential. If we can tap into the tremendous resource that is our brain-power, who knows what we can accomplish?

Here's a personal example of my "not knowing what I didn't know" but thinking that I "knew what I knew." As a child, I was told to wait an hour after eating before going into the ocean to swim. They said that I could get stomach cramps and drown. It was, after all, "common sense." As an adult, when I started heavy swim training and had to swim hard for two to three hours at a time, I found that I couldn't last through a workout without having eaten first. Then I found out that other hardcore swimmers ate before their workouts too. This told me that the eat-swim-drown myth was just that—a myth—and so I revised what I "knew I knew."

It has been more than sixty years since I took college-level philosophy and deductive-logic courses. In that time, I've realized that I could really use a lot of the information I'd gained from those courses, laboring through them as a college student primarily to fulfill graduation requirements. Knowledge that had previously seemed to have little application to my everyday life suddenly was a necessity in sorting valuable facts from mere coincidences.

Years later, in 1969, I was working on my master's degree and then my PhD, and I was sweating through graduate-level courses on statistics and research design. It would be another ten years before I fully grasped the value of being able to evaluate facts, raw data, theories, hypotheses, conjectures, trial-and-error analyses, normal distributions following bell-shaped curves, standard deviations, sampling errors, confidence errors, null hypotheses, highly improbable events, outliers, and just plain old freak accidents.

What little remained in my head after I passed these courses suddenly had applications I'd never dreamed of. It was like discovering a Swiss Army knife in my back pocket when I'd been using my fingernails as a screwdriver and my teeth as pliers. I marveled at how prescient those professors of old were!

I started to see cancer patients and people in general as points on distribution curves. I started thinking in terms of sample sizes and sampling errors. What did it really mean if a fellow athlete had taken the latest electrolyte replacer and gotten his fastest time ever, while another who'd taken the same potion had bonked (hit the wall) so badly that he'd had to drop out of the race? Here was one athlete swearing by this product and here was another cursing it. So what?

When I tried the same electrolyte replacer, I couldn't notice any difference; because of the countless variables involved, it was hard to tell what was going on. Say, for one race, I had gotten an excellent night's sleep the night before but had not had time for my usual pre-race bowl of oatmeal. For the next race, I had been up half the previous night stewing about a problem, had awakened feeling totally exhausted, but had had plenty of time for my usual oatmeal breakfast. Other times, I might have not bothered to put my fancy twelve-spoke racing wheels on or might have decided to wear a tri-suit instead of making clothing changes. As I contemplated the almost-infinite number of variables, I realized how nearly impossible it was to truly *know* anything!

To really scientifically prove a theory, I would need to have two large groups of randomly selected athletes—the first being the experimental group, with one and only one variable, and the other being the control group, with nothing varying. This is the only way to identify the effect of a single variable; otherwise, you don't know which cause had which effect. Can you imagine taking a hundred athletes and, for example, ensuring that they all get eight hours of quality sleep, all have four ounces of oatmeal with blueberries, all wear the same clothing, all use identical equipment, and all have the same level of motivation to win, etc.?

Next, I would have to randomly assign each participant to either the control group or the experimental group. Then I would have to put on a race in which the water conditions were identical for each swimmer, the winds blew at the same speed and in the same direction for each cyclist, and the foot strikes were identical for each runner. Then I would have to look at the finish times of both groups, calculate the mean (arithmetic average) finish time for each group, and determine if the difference, if any, is statistically significant (meaning that it is unlikely that this was a chance variation).

If there was a significant difference between the two groups, I might then be able to conclude that the electrolyte replacer was the variable that caused the difference. But in order to be reliable, the test would have to be replicated by others. Obviously, research like this is rarely, if ever, done.

The Placebo, Nocebo, and Halo Effects

Do we dare consider the confounding factors introduced by the placebo, nocebo, and halo effects? What about the fact that if one of the top triathletes recommends a particular electrolyte replacer, those who believe the hype are prone to the common phenomenon of "getting what you expect to get" (the placebo effect)? What about the opposite, that when told a placebo could cause nausea and vomiting, people find that it does, even though it is inert? That's the nocebo effect at work. Now look at what can happen when an "expert" predicts an event that lies outside of their field of expertise. Whatever happens is frequently interpreted in terms of the prediction, primarily because experts in one area tend to be viewed as figures of authority in other areas as well. This is the halo effect.

Also, in reviewing research papers, you might have a tendency to seize upon those that support your point of view and disregard the others. This is called cherry picking or confirmation bias and can mislead you into supporting a hypothesis that may not be valid.

The mind is so powerful that it's quite possible that if you're told a little magic pill will make you go faster, you may very well go faster. It's almost impossible to eliminate the placebo, halo, or nocebo effects when you are trying different foods, equipment, or psychological processes. Even if you, the subject, don't know whether there's an active ingredient in the pill to make it effective, there's the possibility that the person giving you the pill does and is therefore biased. This is why experiments aren't considered the gold standard—that is, both valid *and* reliable—unless they are double-blinded. This means that neither the subject nor the experimenter knows what's in the pill, which controls for the bias effects, and that subjects need to be randomly assigned for the experiment. You also need to look at who or what is funding the study, which introduces the possibility of bias. Despite this, there are some people who so strongly believe certain things that no amount of evidence to the contrary will shake their faith.

What about the people who think that if X quantity is good, then 2X will be twice as good and 3X will be three times as good? *If I ran my best race on 40 miles a week of running, just think what I could do when I run 80 miles a week or even 120 miles a week*, the logic goes. Indeed, there are people who, incredibly, do run 120 miles or more a week. The problem comes when some of us try to increase our training mileage to these levels and are rewarded only with injury.

To go back to the example of the electrolyte replacer, if our experimental group was significantly faster, we then need to look at the quantity the subjects drank. Let's assume it was 24 ounces. What would have happened if they had drunk only 10 ounces, or conversely, 52 ounces? Now you see that we'd have to run another experiment, holding all other variables the same again, with one control group and three experimental groups. Another question arises: is the fluid-level range of 10, 24, and 52 wide enough to give us conclusions about the *optimum* level? What if 24 ounces is still too much and 52 ounces still too little? What if performance level increases with electrolyte-replacer intake up to 24 ounces and starts to decrease with greater fluid intake? Our experiment with three levels could show that 24 and 52 ounces produce the same results, and we could conclude that performance does not improve with electrolyte-replacer levels of over 24 ounces. You can see why experiments like this are hardly ever done.

The Fallacy of the Truncated Scale

Another factor that must be considered in assessing the value or truthfulness of data is the range or number of data points on the scale. Does the scale go high enough or low enough? Does it completely miss the optimum in the middle? This problem was vividly demonstrated in the Harvard Nurses' Health Study, which examined the diets of 89,494 women and one of the findings of which was that dietary fat did not influence breast cancer rates.[2] The trouble with this conclusion was that *all* the subjects had a high-fat diet, so naturally, there was little, if any, difference in their risks of getting breast cancer! Due to this flaw in the study, a lot of damage continues to be done as women are told not to worry about fat in the diet causing breast cancer. If the data points had gone low enough—with dietary fat down to 10 percent, for example—the results would have been very different.

This fallacy is also misleading the public via advertising campaigns that try to promote the supposedly healthful effects of eating eggs and to reverse the finding that eggs, particular the yolks, are high in cholesterol, thereby raising your total cholesterol levels and elevating your risk of dying of heart disease. Headlines proclaim, "New Research Shows That Eggs Do Not Raise Cholesterol Levels!" The way you set up this "research" is to find subjects who already have very high, saturated levels of cholesterol and to feed them eggs. This, right off the bat, already violates the gold-standard requirement of random subject selection. Sure enough, those subjects would give you the results you want because if your total cholesterol levels are already high, the percentage increase from eating eggs is slight. Research on randomized subjects, however, shows that eating just one egg a day significantly raises the risk of death from heart disease.[3]

Here's another problem generated by a truncated scale. Consider this egregious situation: you read that someone died of a heart attack even though he had a "normal" level of cholesterol of 180 mg/dL—"normal" being in relation to the US population's mean (mathematical average), which is currently under 200 mg/dL. This number, established based on just Americans' cholesterol levels, actually used to be almost 300 mg/dL. If, however, you lower the scale to include China's average level of 120 mg/dL, you can see that the situation is now quite different. He did indeed have a high level of cholesterol.

The same error was repeated in one study with regard to exercise, whose finding was that breast cancer rates were no different between "heavy" and "light" exercisers. The error here was that the researchers' definition of "heavy" was still too light. This is another example of the range of data points not being wide enough—the fallacy of the truncated scale. However, recognizing the problem, the researchers at least concluded that women should exercise anyway. Fortunately, that study has since been withdrawn and replaced with more recent research showing that exercise does help prevent breast cancer.[4]

In addition to the scale of data, researchers must be mindful of individual differences. Some people assume that we are all fundamentally identical, while others assume that we are so different that we can't learn anything from each other. The truth lies in between. Within a broad range, we humans are remarkably similar, but within a narrow range, we are as individual as our fingerprints. As a result, when assessing the outcome of someone else's experimental results, we need to consider whether the results fall within the narrow or the broad range.

It's the similarities we as humans all share that allow blood tests to tell us, for example, whether our iron and cholesterol levels are normal or that allow surgeons to perform the same basic operations such as appendectomies on all of us. After all, it's pretty rare for a surgeon to open someone up and find a real surprise. Of course, there are differences, and that's why we need most of all to keep an open, inquisitive mind and be very careful about drawing conclusions. In addition, a conclusion, once drawn, needs to be held in the light of advancing knowledge. When you find that you are wrong about something, you are on the way to being right.

Compared to What?

You probably frequently see and hear advertisements for prescription drugs that make the claim that drug A—the drug being advertised—reverses certain symptoms better than does drug B. A question that should immediately flash into your mind is, "Drug A compared to what else?" It's possible that both drug A and drug B could have been compared to just an over-the-counter aspirin or perhaps even a placebo.

Alternatively, you might see an ad for a dairy product that claims, "Full-fat dairy is healthier than low-fat dairy." Again, you need to immediately ask yourself, "Compared to what else?" How about to no dairy at all?

By the way, the only two countries that currently allow direct-to-consumer advertising of prescription drugs are the United States and New Zealand. Note that drug advertising results in more costly prescriptions. Few inexpensive drugs are advertised (somebody's got to pay for those ads).

The Blue Zones

How do you account for the fact that three-quarters of the world's population (Africa and Asia) are primarily vegetarian or vegan? You may have heard of the Blue Zones, areas where there are the highest numbers of healthy, physically active, and mentally sharp centenarians. They include Ikaria, Greece; Okinawa, Japan; Sardinia, Italy; Nicoya, Costa Rica; and Loma Linda, California (the only Blue Zone in the US). Inhabitants of the Blue Zones do not eat much animal-based food at all. Yet, incredibly, most Westerners believe that one must consume animal meat and dairy products to be healthy. Say "protein" and most people think of meat. Say "calcium" and they'll think of dairy. This speaks to the power of advertising, money, and lobbying.

This is especially baffling when there is a great deal of scientific evidence that animal foods are responsible for more than 70 percent of all deaths in Western civilization.[5] Nobody wants to die, and yet we keep eating the very foods that cause heart disease, cancer, stroke, diabetes, obesity, osteoporosis, arthritis, dementia, kidney disease, and on and on. After I adopted the new diet and saw first-hand the very positive results it yielded, I wondered what other beliefs I might have that were so firmly entrenched that I dared not question them.

What about Pandemics Like COVID-19?

We are seeing many examples of people not knowing what they don't know, one poignant example being vaccinations. There are some who refuse to get vaccinated because they think the vaccine hasn't been tested enough or because they are misinformed about the vaccine's effectiveness. Then there's the halo effect at play: there are those who are first in line to get the shots because a doctor says they're safe and effective, although that doctor did not participate in the testing. People think they know what they know, but what they "know" may be based on inadequate or wrong information. They are actually operating in the fourth box, not knowing what they don't know. Likewise, most people don't know—and they don't realize that they lack this knowledge—how strong an ally a plant-based vegan diet is in fighting all viruses, including coronavirus and its future variations. There is research showing how a plant-based vegan diet both lowers your risk of getting COVID-19 and, if you do get it, lowers (by 73 percent, to be precise) your risk of experiencing moderate to severe illness as a result. You also enjoy a much lower risk of hospitalization and "long-haul" symptoms.[6]

The essential thing to understand here is that you should get informed about matters regarding your health and be skeptical about graphs and charts. The fitness plan provided in this book involves listening to your body, challenging preconceived notions about what you can or cannot do, not depriving yourself of food or energy, and consequently enjoying a long, healthy life. Remember those Blue Zones!

CHAPTER FOUR

CHANGING ATTITUDES

Have you ever created a resolution to make a major change in your life, then found your willpower crumbling in the face of a lack of support from the people around you and in your environment? One of the reasons why formal education is sometimes ineffective is that although we can change behavior under classroom conditions, as soon as we go back to the "real world," the old behavior resurfaces.

One of the most basic tenets of learning theory is that behavior that is rewarded or positively reinforced will recur and behavior that is not positively reinforced, even negatively reinforced, will drop away or be extinguished. Many people resolve to improve their diet or start an exercise program in order to lose weight, but they soon find themselves falling back into the same old habits of eating the same old foods and not exercising.

What? Me, Change?

The process of changing behavior can be divided into three steps. First, the theory must be learned. Second, the desired behavior must be elicited. Third, it must be rewarded or positively reinforced. All this means is that we need to know what to do, do it, and then want to keep doing it. With this powerful series of steps, we can control our behavior, form new habits, and make ourselves do almost anything we set our minds to.

In my particular case, I was highly motivated to make a dietary change. After all, as I perceived the situation, the penalty for failure was dying of breast cancer. It was the medical equivalent of having a proverbial gun held to my head, forcing me to change or die. My eating habits changed quite literally in two hours: I walked out of Dr. McDougall's office that day committed to a low-fat, whole-food, plant-based vegan diet.

What then amazed me was that I started enjoying food more. The most basic foods, such as oatmeal, fruit, potatoes, carrots, and even broccoli, seemed new. As if for the first time, I tasted the delicious flavors of each of these foods. I didn't need sweeteners, sauces, spices, or the likes to make these foods appetizing. They were already delicious, and I started to appreciate their basic tastes and really relish each of my meals. We now know that our taste buds can quickly change and adapt to new foods. I started loving all leafy greens, especially cilantro, kale, and fennel.

Even at the time, there was already strong evidence that a low-fat, no-oil vegan diet enables people to live longer—another reason why I was highly motivated to adopt it. Then, the reinforcement for my changed eating habits was my rediscovering the good taste of pure, unrefined, whole foods that at the same time were reversing my cancer and high cholesterol, as well as my feeling stronger and more energetic.

You're the One Who's Sick, Not Me!

A major challenge for me was the lack of support from my husband, who saw no application of this diet to his life. You may remember that he told his doctor what I'd said about trying to lower his blood pressure with the new diet and that his doctor assured him, "No, you'll be on these hypertension drugs for the rest of your life." I actually used to have borderline-high blood pressure myself; since my diet change, my blood pressure has been as low as 90/60 for years now. Sadly, today, decades after my husband had that conversation with his doctor, the same arguments are still given when people (and their doctors) are confronted for the first time with information about a low-fat vegan diet. This diet, on the other hand, has helped many people get off their hypertension drugs, as showcased on Dr. McDougall's website (drmcdougall.com).

Had I not had fear as a negative motivator, I'm not sure that I could have stuck with the change. I remember struggling to clear my kitchen of all the offending foods and having to face continuous temptation. My solution was to buy only healthy foods, but then my husband started to bring home the meat, lobster, and butter. We had a side-by-side refrigerator; if you opened the doors, you would see all my foods lined up on one side and his on the other. I must say, though, that after learning about the problems that meat and dairy products cause, I was not only not tempted but even repulsed by the thought of eating any part of a dead animal.

The situation was a little different when I was with friends or in other social environments. Those who knew of my new diet were hesitant to eat in front of me or thought that I would never find anything to eat at restaurants. Things have changed a lot since I became vegan back in 1982, when people could not even pronounce the word "vegan" correctly. Now, there frequently are lots of vegan options for you to try; plus, many restaurant chefs are happy to prepare an off-menu vegan meal.

Ethnic restaurants are probably a fairly safe bet because their menus offer dishes that are the results of generations of people having lived on plant-heavy diets. At Mexican restaurants, for example, you can order side dishes of rice, beans, and corn tortillas. Note that you may have a choice between corn and wheat tortillas. Wheat tortillas are usually made with refined white flour, so go with the corn tortillas. These selections make for an absolutely scrumptious meal, and you'll be amazed at how inexpensively you can eat too!

Chinese, Thai, and Japanese restaurants already serve fairly healthy dishes. Go for the soba (buckwheat) noodles, rice, and vegetables. Indian restaurants are also good bets for healthful eating if you eliminate the dairy. Many of them have a great selection of vegan dishes such as curries and dals. You can ask the chef to prepare your food with no added oils or to skip the monosodium glutamate (MSG) if you're on a low-sodium diet. Again, these meals are usually delicious as well as inexpensive. I have included some internationally inspired recipes at the back of this book for you to try out at home.

Groups Are Powerful Stuff

With regard to exercising, we already know in theory that exercise is good for us and that most of us don't get enough. How do we put into practice our resolutions to exercise more and get to the positive-reinforcement part? One secret I've found is to join a group. This has been a powerful motivator for me. First, a group usually has a leader or coach who provides instruction and encouragement. Second, peer pressure can do wonders in making us want to keep to a task and do it well. As a bonus, the social aspects of group activities are conducive to finding role models, like-minded friends, and in some cases, compatible lovers.

For the first fourteen years, I was a solitary runner. I ran early every morning on the same course, covered the same distance, used the same running style, and did not improve much. Upon finding two running clubs, I joined them both. One was headed by the legendary New Zealander ultra-marathoner Max Telford, who focused on endurance. I started to be able to increase my distance easily thanks to the fast friendships that I was forming, enabling me to run miles painlessly while talking and having fun. My clubmates and I tackled steep hills, bounding and striding up them, laughing all the way. At the end of our workouts, we basked in the good feelings we all had about our training efforts and for each other.

The other club was headed by Johnny Faerber, who was the track coach at the University of Hawaii at the time. This was an all-female group, called Faerber's Flyers, focused on track workouts emphasizing speed. Here I was, at the age of forty-seven, learning a whole new vocabulary with terms such as "400s," "800s," "intervals," and "quarters" and finding out that running around in circles could actually be fun. With the combination of endurance and speed that I honed in my two running clubs, I became a true runner.

I missed a workout only under the direst of emergencies. To illustrate, I recall once getting off a plane after a five-hour flight from Los Angeles to Honolulu and going directly to the track to run with my group! I've done 100-mile around-the-island bicycle rides, gotten off the bike, and moved right on to a track workout. This was in spite of my occasionally being so saddle-sore that I could barely walk.

Swim training in a pool can be so boring that I can hardly ever bring myself to do it alone. Yet with a group, that all changes. To keep yourself motivated, swim in lanes with timers to indicate your progress. Coaches are a necessity here, because swim technique is critical to racing fast, and swim form deteriorates rapidly under fatigue. Even when I'm not tired, it seems that I need constant reminders to keep my elbows high. More on this later.

The bike rides I mentioned above, I would never have undertaken alone. In the first place, I always do long rides using the buddy system. It is the safest thing to do and would immediately prove useful in case of accident or mechanical failure. Secondly, a boring ride is transformed into something joyous when you're riding with compatible people. I found the experiences shared on these group rides so reinforcing that I was hooked on them even when I was not training. Others must have as well since we always had a nice, large, and willing group.

As a fringe benefit, we saw some of the most glorious sights in the world on our rides. In Hawaii, on the island of Oahu, you can start out by climbing over Diamond Head, go past Hanauma Bay, and scream downhill to Sandy Beach to see some of the most beautiful rocky seacoasts on the island. On clear mornings, you might be able to see all the way to the outer islands of Molokai and, rarely, even Maui and Lanai. These experiences are so exciting that I wish I could share them with the whole world!

As you can probably tell, I'm something of a health evangelist. I'm on a mission to try to get people out onto the roads or into the ocean, just as I implore them to try eating a diet of 100 percent plant foods, for just twenty-one days at first. Many said they'd try getting out there, loved it, and are still out there. A few tried it, got away from it, intended to get back to it, and somehow never quite did, but still loved the idea. Some said they'd tried it and felt weak or lacked energy, maybe even gained weight, so they went back to being sedentary and eating meat. (On a related note, this points to the fact that there are many ways to eat a vegan diet—indeed, there are "junk-food vegans"—and you do need to do it right.) Then there are those who refuse to even *try*. The people in the first two groups are your athletic supporters. Those in the other groups obviously need some real motivation and education, so there is still hope!

Surround yourself with athletic supporters and you won't have any problem maintaining a healthy and fun diet and exercise program. Given the right circumstances, changing attitudes can lead to radical transformation!

CHAPTER FIVE

CHANGING YOUR DIET

When I made the switch to a whole-food, plant-based, low-fat vegan diet, I found that for the first time in my life, my bowels functioned the way they were supposed to. In previous years, I could not eat very much for fear of gaining weight. As a result, I was always hungry and had pellet–sized stools, which were brought forth only under great strain. I was told by physicians and thus thought that two or three bowel movements a *week* were probably normal for me. The day after I changed my diet, I discovered what "normal" is supposed to be! In fact, when I give talks on how I reversed my cancer, often the first question is, "How soon did the diet start working?" to which I would smile and say, "The next morning!" (And then I wait for folks to get it.)

It is obvious from all the TV, radio, magazine, and other ads that constipation and hemorrhoids are common among Americans. Had I weighed and measured the stools of people from other cultures, as Sir Denis Burkitt, MD did in Africa, I would have found out that most of these people had large, bulky, soft stools that moved effortlessly and frequently and had a transit time (time of travel from mouth to anus) of eight hours or less, as opposed to the thirty-six to fifty-two hours seen in England, where Sir Denis carried out his groundbreaking research, and probably in the US as well.[1] I would have also found out that there were entire societies without colon cancer or a single case of hemorrhoids—indeed, they would not even know what hemorrhoids were.

No longer was I plagued with worry about being able to move my bowels before a race or having to make an emergency pit stop during it. I learned that a proper diet normalizes the intestinal tract and its microbiome—all the good-guy bugs including bacteria and viruses inhabiting your colon that help keep you healthy. I get to relearn this lesson occasionally, usually when I am traveling and not able to get my usual amount of fiber.

The Importance of Fiber

Research on the human gut has exploded in the past ten years. We now know that our gut microbiome thrives on high-fiber foods, with our "good bacteria" digesting the fiber to produce short-chain fatty acids (SCFAs) to nourish our colon cells and boost our immune system. Indeed, dietary fiber is the only way we can get SCFAs. We cannot produce them ourselves, yet they are crucial for good gut and immune-system health, helping to prevent leaky gut syndrome, autoimmune disease, and many other chronic illnesses.

Even more amazing to me was the discovery that each plant, even each unique variety of the same species, has its own microbiome. Perhaps unsurprisingly, the more varied the plant foods in your diet, the more diverse the "good bugs" in your own microbiome too. About 70 percent of your immune system is in the cells lining your gut. Whole plant foods are the only source of fiber; animal foods have no fiber, absolutely none. I once had a back-and-forth with a medical doctor who thought that the tendons in animals are made of fiber. He was obviously a victim of the nutrition-education deficiency that prevails in most medical schools. You also need to know that highly refined and processed foods have lost most of their fiber. We need to really appreciate how a whole-food, plant-based diet dovetails so beautifully with our gut microbiome to boost our immune system![2]

More Fiber, Please!

Diverticulosis is another affliction that is common in this country and rare in countries with low-fat, high-fiber diets. Diverticula are little outpouchings that occur in the intestines when the muscles involved in peristaltic movements (muscular contractions that move food through the GI tract) do not have enough bulk to "grab." It's rather like inflating a balloon with weak spots. The weak spots in the intestines bulge out and form little pockets. Diverticula are prone to irritation, inflammation, and infection and can be very painful. When this happens, the condition is called diverticulitis, and like so many other common diseases in the US, it's preventable by a high-fiber diet.

Why Whole Foods?

In this regard, there are two sometimes-controversial issues: sugar and juicing. Some people find these topics confusing partly because they do not fully understand the terminology. First of all, why do some people say, "Sugar is bad, so don't eat fruit"? The problem is that there are too many different definitions of sugar. There are actually over two hundred different names for different types of sugars. It's no wonder people get confused!

Healthy vs. Refined Sweeteners

The white sugar found in sugar bowls did start as a whole food—as beet, corn, or sugar cane that was then heavily processed and refined to turn into the white substance people are familiar with. It's what's commonly used to sweeten beverages, such as soda and coffee, and as an ingredient called for by recipes of decadent desserts such as cakes, pies, cookies, and puddings. It adds no nutritional value whatsoever, only so-called "empty calories."

The problem with refined sweeteners, though they may start as whole foods—again, primarily beets, sugar cane, and corn—is that they end up as a sugar called fructose. From fructose are derived almost all of the types of sugar you'll encounter on food labels, such as sucrose, maltose, dextrose, galactose, and high fructose corn syrup. Any sugar whose name ends with -ose, you typically want to avoid; it is one of the highly refined, so-called "bad carbs" and "bad sugars" that have high glycemic indexes, meaning that they spike your blood sugar levels and can lead to diabetes when coupled with a high-fat diet.

Stevia powder is a healthy sweetener as it is just the ground-up dried leaves of the stevia plant with no added fillers. It is so sweet that all you have to add is less than one-sixteenth of a teaspoon. Alternatively, I've actually found that one of the best sweeteners is the lowly prune. It is truly a multitasker in that it helps the bowels and is good for the bones as well; plus, prunes are healthier and cheaper than dates. Try throwing a few into your next smoothie. If the idea sounds far-fetched because you've usually seen only dates called for in recipes, I promise you that prunes can make a great-tasting sweetener.

Blood sugar, called glucose, is what the body gets from digesting food, specifically carbohydrates. "Good sugars" come contained in whole foods such as fruits and starchy vegetables. These include corn, peas, squash, potatoes, and yams, which all have lower glycemic indexes, meaning that they don't spike your blood sugar. The sugar from these sources is slowly digested, some of which is in the form of long-chain complex sugars called starch. Starch is another form of the "good sugars." Dr. McDougall says that we are all really "starchivores" and evolved as such. One need only look at how some of the healthiest populations maintain starch-based diets and have done so for many generations.

Unfortunately, starches have gotten a bad rap due to the prevalent myth that they make you fat. Actually, it's the fat, not the starches, you eat that makes you fat. Some people are told not to eat white potatoes partly because of the mistaken belief that they spike blood sugar levels. They are healthy; it's the butter, gravy, and bacon bits added to mashed or baked potatoes that make them unhealthy. Potatoes contain both simple and complex carbohydrates (starches) that the body breaks down into glucose through a slow absorption process, generating a more gradual, continuous flow of energy. These are the "good carbs" that make up around 80 percent of the calories in a healthy diet, the remainder being divided evenly between protein and fat. Sadly, healthy populations who have traditionally eaten in ways similar to this are feeling the effects of their diets being westernized.

What's Wrong with Juicing?

When you eat the whole fruit and not just its juice, you get a large dose of fiber, which slows down the absorption of sugar so that there's no spike in your blood sugar levels, which, as mentioned before, is important in helping to prevent diabetes. When you juice a fruit, it is no longer a whole food and no longer needs chewing, which is the first step in digestion; because the juice has no fiber, it also spikes blood sugar levels just like the "bad sugars" do. Some people want to juice foods like carrots, apples, beets, celery, or leafy greens because that way, they can get a concentrated source of nutrients, but this comes with the loss of all that healthy fiber. Generally speaking, a whole-food, plant-based diet provides all the nutrients and fiber you need and, with a slow, steady absorption rate, also sustains you over the long haul. More of something isn't necessarily better and can actually be counterproductive.

What about Lignans?

Lignans are compounds that are found in certain plants and that have a chemical structure very similar to the hormone estrogen. They are thus called phytoestrogens (*phyto* meaning "plant"). They can attach themselves to estrogen receptor sites, blocking them and thereby reducing the risk of breast cancer by keeping estrogen levels low. Studies have shown that a higher intake of lignans, the main phytoestrogen in flaxseeds, is associated with a lower risk of breast cancer. Just a single teaspoon of ground flaxseeds may double your total daily intake of lignans. Less abundant sources of lignans include vegetables, cereal grains, legumes, and beans.

Moreover, for women who have been diagnosed with breast cancer, higher lignans in the diet are associated with a less aggressive cancer and a longer survival time—just another one of the many reasons to eat a whole-food, plant-based diet! A number of studies supporting the above are cited by Michael Greger, MD on his website (nutritionfacts.org).

But I'll Starve to Death!

Amazingly, another preventable side effect of dieting so many people in this country suffer from is constant hunger, caused by there being not enough food in the stomach. Many people try to control their weight by just eating less, via "portion control" or the "push away from the table" method, and therefore suffer from those pangs of hunger. The problem is that these methods don't work. Even if you manage to lose a few pounds, once you go back to your old way of eating, you would gain all the weight back and then some. Compare the difference between a hundred calories of oil (one tablespoon) and a hundred calories of potato (a large one). Which do you think will do a better job of filling you up?

Double or Even Triple Your Pleasure!

What most people don't know is that they can actually eat two to three times more food (quantity-wise) and still lose weight! Most plant foods are low in calories, so you can fill up and feel satisfied on this program. If you need to lose weight, the exceptions would be nuts, seeds, avocados, olives, and coco-nuts, which would need to be limited because they are quite high in fat.

Since hunger is one of the most powerful drives, most people who try to deprive themselves will soon succumb and will frequently go overboard once they decide, "To heck with it." Their bodies compensate for the period of "starvation" by storing extra calories as body fat. Sensing that food is once again plentiful and they are no longer at risk of going hungry, their bodies start restoring (*re-storing*, literally) fat reserves. The human body does this as a survival mechanism to get ready for the next bout of scarcity. The bad news is that with practice, it gets more efficient at laying in fat stores, and one ends up with a higher body-fat percentage and a lower lean body mass. This means that there is less muscle with which to burn up calories—one reason why the body puts lost fat back on more easily. Then come the pangs of guilt and new resolutions, and the cycle begins again.

This is why exercise is so important: it combats your tendency to lose muscle when you're not using it; it may even help you gain muscle. It is also why low-calorie diets don't work. Whenever you start restricting your food intake, you are up against the most powerful of survival mechanisms. If people only knew that they can eat as much as they want, until they are completely satisfied, and that they can even lose weight on such a plan, wouldn't you wonder why they wouldn't all do it? Boy, I sure would!

I have all of my favorite foods first thing in the morning: oatmeal with blueberries, a heaping teaspoon of 100% organic cocoa powder, a tiny bit of stevia as sweetener, and some leafy greens. The last ingredient may sound a little strange, but just try it! The first time I tried greens with my breakfast was when I worked at the 1988 Seoul Olympics and got to eat with all the athletes in the Olympic Village in Seoul, South Korea. Each country had a booth with its own customary meals. Because I was around so many Asian athletes, many of whom ate greens in the form of seaweed for breakfast, I decided to try it and liked it. I began to try other greens such as kale, edible hibiscus, and even cabbage. Since I consider greens the gold standard of nutrition, I try to get them in as often as possible, even at breakfast to start off each day. The spruced-up oatmeal I have for breakfast is quite filling and enough to sustain me throughout a good early-morning workout or race.

My lunches and dinners are usually centered on starches. Regular white potatoes, sweet potatoes, purple sweet potatoes, and yams can be sliced and microwaved for five to ten minutes for nearly instant satisfaction. There is a suggested weeklong menu, with recipes, provided at the back of this book.

I usually end supper with a dessert of an apple and some goji berries. Goji berries are high in lutein and zeaxanthin, which are needed for a healthy macula and good eyesight.

I have been eating like this for over forty years. What I've found is that plain, whole, unprocessed foods can taste great. Admittedly, I made the change literally under threat of death. But the rediscovery of the wholesome, good taste of pure, plain, unadulterated foods was more than a pleasant surprise.

But What Does It Do for Energy?

I found my energy levels soaring! Wouldn't you agree that this would have to be the case in order for me to train for an event like the Ironman triathlon? I rarely took a day off from training, and when I did, it was usually from the press of other business. I rarely had to cut short a workout, and when I did, it was most frequently from running out of time. I'd then say to myself, "Just one more lap," or, "Just one more mile."

I slept like a rock, as they say, and rarely suffered from any kind of depression or moodiness. The most frequent comment I heard from my coaches and friends was that I raced too much. I was especially delighted to hear this from "youngsters"—people twenty to thirty years younger than me. I really did race a lot, as I've detailed in an earlier chapter. I'd been doing on average fifty races a year ever since my diagnosis, and I hit a new high of sixty-three races in 1997. (I had turned sixty-four years of age that year and was actually on my way to sixty-four races in 1998 when I was hit by a truck while training on my bike. More on that later.) That works out to at least one race almost every weekend, all year round. I would have done more except that most of the races started at the same time, 7 a.m. on Sunday morning!

There was one time when I participated in three races in a single weekend. There was a sunset "fun run" on Friday evening, then there was a 5K race and a sprint triathlon, both on Sunday morning. The 5K race started at 7 a.m.; I finished it by 7:20 a.m., got into my car parked near the finish line, drove to Kailua on the other side of the island, made the

8 a.m. start, and did the triathlon. I got first place in both events, and by coincidence, the next morning, the results were posted next to each other on the paper's sports page. I got a call from the sports editor asking how this was possible, so I explained the planning involved. I suppose it was enough of a story that he turned it into an article.

I also completed three marathons in three weeks—not that I planned it that way. I was entered in two marathons that were two weeks apart, allowing for one week's recovery time in between, which I knew was adequate. Then a dear friend who had signed up for a marathon right in between the two asked me if I would run with her for moral support. How could I say "no"?

But Where Do You Get Your _____ (Fill in the Blank)?

I cite all of this as evidence that a whole-food, plant-based, low-fat vegan diet can't be all that lacking in total calories, protein, essential fatty acids, vitamins, minerals (such as calcium), and all the other factors that detractors usually quote. The question that I hear the most often from people is, "Where do you get your protein?" followed by, "Where do you get your calcium?" These are covered below.

First, when it comes to calories, they all come from one of three macronutrients—carbohydrates, protein, and fat. The ideal diet should consist of approximately 10 percent protein and 10 percent fat, with the remaining and highest percentage coming from carbohydrates.

Carbohydrates

The preferred source of energy for your muscles and your brain is glucose, which comes only from carbohydrates. The best source of carbohydrates is plant foods; in fact, animal foods provide few, if any, carbohydrates. Getting enough calories is a matter of balancing calorie-dense foods such as whole grains, starches, and dried fruit with low–caloric-density foods such as leafy greens. This is how to control weight loss and weight gain.

What about carbo-loading? Carbo-loading is a technique used by some athletes to increase the proportion of glucose that is converted to glycogen, the form of sugar that your muscles use and that derives from carbohydrates.

During a hard training bout or a race, you use up your glycogen. You then need to replace it by eating carbohydrates. If you are eating a whole-food, plant-based diet, you don't need to do anything differently since you are essentially carbo-loading every day. As a result, you are always ready for anything—training or a competition in almost any sport.

Protein

Ask any doctor if they have ever seen a case of protein deficiency, and they will have to say they have not. In fact, there is no way that you can be deficient in protein as long as you are eating enough calories from whole plant foods. Protein is made of up of amino acids, which get broken down during digestion and which your circulatory system then distributes throughout your body to wherever they are needed. There are nine essential amino acids, and most vegetables and grains contain adequate amounts of all of these essential amino acids. Some people will have to go back and read that sentence again, but it's true. Even fruit has some protein; there are quite a few long-term, healthy fruitarians. In the popular press, I still frequently find perpetuated the myth that you need animal protein for a "complete" protein source, that you need to "combine" proteins to get all the essential amino acids, or that soy beans are the only complete plant protein. None of this is true, which becomes obvious when you look up tables (say, on the USDA's official website, usda.gov) showing the essential-amino-acid content in foods such as rice, potatoes, corn, oats, broccoli, taro, and green leafy vegetables. Again, these foods possess all of the essential amino acids, and if eaten in sufficient quantity to satisfy caloric needs, they will satisfy our protein needs.

But don't some people—athletes, bodybuilders, and the elderly, for example—need more protein in their diet? It's as if people believe that when eaten, protein gets magically transformed into muscle—more protein equals more muscle. Actually, you make your muscles stronger and larger by increasing the work that they do. Then, when your muscles have to work more, you burn more calories, your appetite increases, and by eating more, you automatically get more protein. Just popping protein pills isn't going to do it.

Despite its obsession with this macronutrient, Western society has no problem getting enough protein—quite the opposite. It is actually getting too much protein. And if that protein is of animal origin, you put yourself at risk for osteoporosis, kidney failure, arthritis, erectile dysfunction, dementia, and respiratory problems (such as asthma, allergies, mucous formation, and sinusitis). Sadly, most people aren't told this and doctors aren't taught this in medical schools, although this is starting to change. There is now a specialty called lifestyle medicine that covers nutrition.

Fat

When the subject of low-fat diets comes up, people frequently say, "But we need fat in our diet." Yes, indeed, we do need some fat in our diet, but it needs to be the "good fats," mainly the omega-3 fatty acids. These are the essential fatty acids, which we get from almost every whole food we eat. For example, lettuce is 13 percent fat, celery 6 percent fat, and oatmeal 16 percent fat. The problem is not getting too little fat but getting too much and, usually, the wrong kinds—saturated fats, trans-fats, and the omega-6 fatty acids.

Low-fat also means no added vegetable oil or margarine. You don't need it, and by adding it, you might just raise your dietary-fat percentage to levels at which heart disease and cancer, especially breast cancer, become more prominent risks. Margarine is not a good substitute for butter for a number of reasons. Although margarine itself has no cholesterol, the oils it contains have to be hydrogenated to make it solid at room temperature and the oil molecules have to be converted to trans-fatty acids, a key component of hardened vegetable oils. It is this formation of trans-fatty acids that alters the structure of fat molecules and raises your total cholesterol levels. Consuming margarine blocks the action of prostaglandins, which help to lower blood pressure and increase the removal of excess sodium from your body.[3] In addition, all fats—margarine and vegetable oils included—seem to increase the incidence of all types of cancer. In sum, it seems not to matter whether the fat is saturated, monounsaturated, or polyunsaturated. It's best to keep your fat percentage as low as possible.

In 2005, Dr. T. Colin Campbell published his first book, *The China Study*, which presents his finding that the lower the dietary-fat intake (down to 5 percent of total calories), the healthier the people. Incidentally, his research also showed that casein, a protein in dairy, can turn cancer "on and off" like a light switch. The research was done on rats, since researchers would not be allowed to conduct this type of experimentation on humans, but there is reason to believe the same mechanism would apply to us.[4] On a related note, vegans value the humane treatment of *all* animals, not just those we call "pets," and believe it's also unethical to experiment on animals. Not only does research on animals inflict immense cruelty on the animals, but this research is frequently misleading and useless.

Calcium

Another question that frequently comes up is where you would get your calcium if you don't consume dairy products. The answer is that you get your calcium from the same sources that cows, horses, elephants, and rhinos get theirs—plant foods, primarily greens. In any case, the problem is usually not one of a calcium deficiency but one of an excess of protein and amino acids. When you eat too much acidic protein, your body has to buffer all that acid, which it does with calcium—a base (meaning it's alkaline)—from your bones.

Supplements

B_{12} is the only vitamin that you need to supplement to make sure you get enough of because neither plants nor animals produce it. It is produced by bacteria. And since our food is routinely washed and we rarely go out to the garden, pull up a carrot, and eat it as is, it turns out that even people who are not vegan may also have low levels of B_{12} and should take a supplement. Taking a blood test is the surest way to see if you have an adequate amount of B_{12}. Either of the two forms commonly found in supplements, methylcobalamin and cyanocobalamin, will work. As for vitamin D, adequate sun exposure is necessary. Vitamin D deficiencies in most people are due to not spending enough time in the sun to get an adequate amount of exposure, especially if they live at higher latitudes.

Lots of people feel so much better eating a low-fat, whole-food, plant-based diet that most who have switched would never go back to their old ways. They are no longer ever tempted to eat health-destroying foods and say they wish they'd made the change a long time ago. For those who still miss any animal-based food, there are whole recipe books available offering tasty vegan versions of classic dishes that when compared with the animal-based versions, taste no different according to some. Stick to whole foods as much as possible and avoid the highly processed, highly refined varieties of "fake" meats, such as those that contain soy protein isolates. (By comparison, whole soy beans and whole soy products are actually very healthy.) What I have found is that this dietary program actually encourages an exercise program. You do more exercise because you have so much more energy and feel so good afterwards!

The Secret to Health and Fitness

I remember coming out of the water one day, having just completed a two-mile swim, with a revelation of sorts. The "secret" to health and fitness is *what* you put in your body and *how* you move it around. The idea should be to input nothing but good food and to aid in your body's circulation of that good food with lots of exercise. It all seemed so simple. Every one of the trillions of cells in your body has three requirements: nutrients, oxygen, and the removal of waste products. A proper diet takes care of the first and exercise takes care of the second and third!

The Growing Problem of Obesity

There are people who go from one fad diet to another, one commercial weight-loss program to another, with no lasting results. Some are so desperate that they resort to bariatric surgery, such as bypass surgery or gastric sleeve surgery, which alters the gastrointestinal tract so as to limit the absorption of calories. These people have spent literally thousands of dollars and still have fat, sick bodies.

The issue for many people is cosmetic. This is best illustrated by the popularity of liposuction surgery. For these people, their major motivator is obviously not health but aesthetics. This is not to downplay the importance of feeling good about how you look, which no doubt plays a major role in your self-esteem. You just need to know that you can have a beautiful, sexy body by adopting a lifestyle that is conducive to it.

Since so many people will, at some time in life, go on one of the new diabetes drugs, resort to fasting or intermittent fasting, or follow a calorie-reduction diet to try to lose weight, it's important to reiterate why these methods don't work. As soon as you get off the pills or the diet and go back to the way of eating that caused the problem in the first place, you'll likely regain all of the lost weight and then some, because your body will have learned how to deposit fat more efficiently.

Okay, Limit Your Oxygen!

Imagine a weight-loss center saying to you: "Okay, we're going to put you on a restricted oxygen diet. You can only take three-quarters of your normal breath each time for the next week. Check back in with us afterwards, and we'll see how you're doing."

Since you're all motivated, and especially since you've paid a lot of money, you charge out the door determined to follow the instructions. How successful do you think you will be? Sure, you can hold your breath for a couple of minutes, but the drive to breathe will always prevail.

You're dealing with a very similar situation when you tell people that they can eat only 75 percent of what they normally eat. They start obsessing about hot fudge sundaes, chocolate candy bars, and banana splits. They probably could stick to the 75 percent program for a little while and maybe lose some weight along the way, but not for very long. As soon as they go off the diet, they will, as we learned earlier, regain that lost weight and then some!

Here's another example. Try to deprive yourself of sleep. Sure, you might be able to stay up for one, two, maybe even up to ten nights, but the drive to sleep will always prevail. After only a day or two, your brain will be grabbing bits of microsleep.

There's no way to beat the system. We humans have, for the most part, pretty strong survival mechanisms. Even if your "willpower" lasts long enough for you to get your weight down, it will not stay down once you go back to your old eating habits. Most people will soon chuck the whole idea and binge to make up for lost calories. That's why the whole system of dieting fails, whether it's a self-imposed, medical, or commercial program. (You can read more about obesity and weight control in chapter 7.)

You can let your appetite be your guide as long as you're eating low–caloric-density foods, just as you let your body breathe and sleep as much as it needs to. It eventually will, anyway! None of this is within your control. What you can control, however, is what foods you choose to put in your body.

In order to lose weight and keep it lost, you must make a lifestyle change, and this lifestyle change must include a shift to a whole-plant-food, low-fat diet, along with an adequate amount of exercise. Lately, best-selling books on dieting that promote high-protein diets such as the Paleo and keto diets have been getting a lot of press. Unfortunately, low-carb and high-protein or high-fat diets don't work for long and even can be dangerous. Unbeknownst to the people who follow these diets, their health is severely compromised in the long run.

The other part of the problem is that people are drawn to any diet that claims it's okay to eat some animal foods (such as chicken or especially fish), which they think would be too difficult for them to give up entirely. If this is you, you could use faux-meat products such as vegan burgers and vegan fish sticks as "transitional" foods as you work on adopting a healthier lifestyle.

There are a couple of diets that get closer to being healthy, such as the DASH (Dietary Approach to Stop Hypertension) and Mediterranean diets, but they still miss the mark because they include fish and oil. Books that promote these almost-healthy diets are not telling the truth about the folks who are successfully living on a low-fat, whole-food, plant-based vegan diet. A healthy vegan diet does work, and there are millions here to attest to that fact. Of course, less optimal vegan diets exist, but you should avoid the many refined, junk-food vegan products that are on the market now or at least limit them to just an occasional treat.

A weight-control program begins with your grocery shopping. A good rule to follow is to shop only at the edges of the store. Depending, of course, on the store's layout, you'll probably find the produce section on one end and bakery goods on another. Go "hog wild" with the vegetables, fruits, and whole grains!

If It Has a Face or a Label, Don't Eat It!

Here's a little rule of thumb: if a food comes from any being with a face, eyes that could look back at you, or a mom and a dad, don't eat it. I'll never forget the day when I said this in a lecture, someone in the audience shouted out, "Or if it poops!" and we all cracked up. Here's the thing: if something fits that criterion, it also has muscles. The muscles are what you would consume, and all muscles have cholesterol and saturated fat. These two substances cause major damage to your body, clogging your circulatory system and your kidneys and suppressing your immune system. Excess cholesterol leads to heart disease and stroke, saturated fat to cancer. These are the top, most common causes of death in the US. That's why I promote a vegan diet—no animal products whatsoever.

My other rule to not eat foods that come with a label came about after I heard so many admonitions to read food labels—to see the list of all that had been added to a product. Labels are found on foods that come in boxes, cans, tins, or jars. The rule is: if it has a label, don't eat it, or at least be very suspicious! Now, that may sound a little extreme, but if it has a label, and especially if you can't pronounce all the ingredients, this usually means that it's been processed (i.e., has had something removed or added, often chemicals or preservatives). Either way, you lose.

Stick to whole foods and you can't go wrong. All you have to do is look at the animal kingdom and see which animals are vegan. Tortoises are the longest-living animal, with a lifespan of over a hundred years. Gorillas are the strongest. Elephants are the largest. These plant-eating animals, by the way, live much longer than meat-eating animals do—more than twice as long, to be exact. For example, an elephant's lifespan is sixty-five years, compared to a tiger's, which is eight to ten years.

But You Do Eat Fish, Don't You?

I hear this question all the time, and then I see people's shocked expressions that follow my emphatic, "No, absolutely not!"

Predictably, the response is, "But what's wrong with fish?" Well, there's a lot that's wrong with fish.

We know that too much animal protein increases your risk of kidney disease and osteoporosis (see more in chapter 15); fish qualifies as a concentrated source of animal protein. Since most people get too much protein, we don't need fish for that reason. What about the omega-3 fatty acids in fish oil that are supposed to be so good for you? Well, if you are eating a diet with lots of leafy green vegetables, you get omega-3 fatty acids from the same source that fish do—plants! (Fish get their omega-3s from seaweed or algae since no animal, including fish, can make them.) In addition, you can boost your omega-3s with some ground flaxseeds or chia seeds.

The flesh of fish is also one of the most contaminated of foods. Even fish found in open oceans are exposed to pesticides, herbicides, microplastics, and heavy metals such as mercury, lead, cadmium, and arsenic. They are also sources of hepatitis, polio, *E. coli*, salmonella, ciguatera poisoning, and an array of parasites such as *Anisakis simplex* (a gastrointestinal worm) and *Clonorchis sinensis* (a liver fluke).[5] Farmed fish are even worse. Crowded into a polluted, antibiotic-laden fecal soup, they are not the answer to our depleting the ocean's fish stocks.

As you can see, there are many reasons to eat a plant-based diet and no reason not to. It's even ideal for children and pregnant people. Besides, the food tastes delicious and makes you feel fabulous. What else could you ask for from a diet?

Getting Started: Food Tips and Recipes

Setting up your kitchen is much easier on this program. The following kitchen tools are useful: paring and chopping knives, a chopping block, pots and pans in various sizes (avoid aluminum ones and ones with Teflon nonstick coating), baking dishes, cooking spoons, a colander, a grater, measuring cups and spoons, mixing bowls, pizza pans, a soup ladle, and sprouting jars and lids. I also cannot get along without my Vitamix blender, slow-cooker, and electric wok, which allows me to whip up an almost infinite variety of no-oil stir-fry dishes. Instead of oil, use water, vegan broth, balsamic vinegar, or low-sodium soy sauce to sauté. Or get an air-fryer.

Staple foods to keep on hand are a variety of whole grains (oats, wheat berries, rye, buckwheat, millet, etc.), vegetables (potatoes, yams, carrots, celery, cabbage, tomatoes, broccoli, etc.), fruit (bananas, mangoes, oranges, apples, berries, melons, prunes, raisins, etc.), and spices (cinnamon, basil, chili powder, cumin, mustard, oregano, sage, thyme, turmeric, rosemary, etc.). With these foods always stocked up, you can make a variety of healthful, delicious meals.

The following are guidelines for beverages, meals, snacks, desserts, and clean-up. At the end of this book is a suggested seven-day meal plan, along with supporting recipes.

Beverages: The best drink in the world is nature's purest—water. First thing in the morning, I have two large glasses of water, followed by a mug of coffee as I'm doing my morning exercise—my physical therapy routines. I didn't used to drink coffee until I read research showing that three to five cups a day can lower rates of dementia.[6]

An alternative—or an addition—to coffee is a tablespoon of organic blackstrap molasses mixed in with a cup of hot water. Not only is this beverage stimulant-free, but it also gives you a good percentage of the day's requirement of iron, calcium, magnesium, and other minerals. Granted, it is not a whole food—quite the opposite. It is actually a concentrated source of all the minerals from the sugar cane plant, removed in the refining process.

Another alternative is green tea, preferably organic. Next to water, tea is the most widely consumed beverage in the world. Along with white tea, green tea is the least processed; it also has the lowest level of caffeine and the highest levels of antioxidants. Moreover, green-tea consumption has been linked to improved memory and lower rates of Alzheimer's disease.[7]

Another beverage you can keep on hand in the refrigerator is lemonade—the old-fashioned kind. Squeeze half a lemon into a half-gallon jug of water and add stevia as a sweetener—just enough to take the edge off. This is a wonderful, healthy thirst-quencher that can help keep your appetite under control too, if you're trying to lose weight.

Breakfast: A very popular breakfast consists of a bowl of oatmeal, with the oats either soaked overnight and cooked or perhaps not even cooked, since oats can be eaten raw too. It does not matter whether it's regular or quick-cooking oats; quick-cooking oats are just rolled thinner. (Just avoid those little packets of instant oatmeal, which is sweetened with sugar.) Add a cup of blueberries, and to further boost the nutritional value, add some leafy greens, as mentioned earlier.

For special breakfasts, you can make healthy whole-grain, no-oil pancakes or waffles. For toppings, add applesauce or fruit purée. Naturally, skip the butter or margarine as it's not at all necessary for a satisfying taste once you get used to the delicious flavors of the other ingredients.

This selection also works for breakfasts eaten out. You can almost always find oatmeal and pancakes on the menu. Some of the more health-conscious restaurants make whole-wheat or buckwheat pancakes, which, of course, are better for you than the standard white-flour-mix ones. Again, leave out the butter or margarine. While others may be raising their cholesterol and fat levels with bacon-and-eggs breakfasts, you will be doing your body a huge favor and enjoying your breakfast just as much or probably more.

Lunches: Your mid-day meal can be any one of many different selections. Some possibilities include: baked or microwaved potatoes with carrot and celery sticks, whole-grain pita bread stuffed with sliced mixed vegetables, quinoa mixed with frozen succotash, and even leftovers from the night before. A healthy brown-bag lunch could be a whole-wheat bagel with a banana, an orange, or an apple.

Dinners: These are some healthy suggestions that most people, even children, like:

- Spaghetti made with whole-wheat pasta and marinara sauce consisting of tomato paste, onions, garlic, bell peppers, broccoli florets, and seasonings. The broccoli can fool people into thinking you've got meatballs, and you can tell kids these are "baby trees"!
- Chili-non-con-carne made with white, black, pinto, and/or kidney beans, tomato sauce, onions, garlic, bell pepper, whole kernel corn, and lots of chili powder, assuming you like it hot!
- Pizza made with a whole-grain crust covered with a tomato-based sauce, with chopped green onions, red onions, bell peppers, mushrooms, and alfalfa or broccoli sprouts. For an "instant" crust, use pita bread or chapatis.

One of the biggest advantages of eating this way is that you can modify almost any of your old favorite dishes. Just skip the animal products, fats, and oils. When you skip meat, increase the veggies. When you skip oils, increase the water. If you want to stir-fry or sauté anything, do it with water, vegan broth, balsamic vinegar, or low-sodium soy sauce. It works very well.

Go to some of the ethnic grocery stores to get ideas for some really interesting foods. For example, Asian grocery stores in your neighborhood sell many different types of Asian foods such as water chestnuts, bamboo shoots, gobo root, a wide variety of Chinese cabbages, and red, black, and brown rice, although you'll need to check where they are grown. Many soils have been contaminated with arsenic, unfortunately.

You can also make your main dish a large salad—but certainly not the usual iceberg lettuce with a slice of tomato. It can be a large, healthy selection of veggies such as cherry tomatoes, bell peppers, cucumbers, celery, broccoli, red onions, and radishes. While browsing through the produce section, look at the variety of lettuces, cabbages, and other greens, especially some of the newer varieties. They are usually inexpensive, especially relative to meat, and add such interesting combinations of colors and textures to your meal. You can also add snow peas, bean sprouts, corn, okra, eggplant, or whatever you see that looks good. Get creative with some of the gourmet greens now available. Just don't ruin a great salad with a commercial high-fat salad dressing.

With regard to salad dressings, I long ago decided to skip them. I love the taste of salads just plain. For those who can't handle that, try a dressing of Dijon mustard, Italian spices, nutritional yeast, a vinegar such as balsamic, apple cider, or rice vinegar, minced garlic or garlic powder, and lemon juice. There are also lots of commercial vegan, no-oil salad dressings on the market now.

Snacks: Almost any fruit, celery or carrot sticks, sweet potatoes, or almost any leftovers. If you keep the high-fat foods out of the house, they can't tempt you. Remember: with this way of eating, you can eat a lot and often, all the while getting to and easily maintaining an ideal body weight.

Desserts: To satisfy that sweet tooth and still have a healthy dessert, try any of the many varieties of fruit in season. If that's not an option, frozen fruit, such as organic strawberries, blueberries, cherries, pineapple, and even dragon fruit, is always a possibility. If you want a special treat, you can throw some peeled, frozen bananas into a blender for a delicious "nice cream." Adding frozen strawberries or any other fruit can give you any number of different flavored "nice creams."

Cost: One last point concerns expense. You will be amazed by how little your food will cost on this program. Nobody believes me when I talk about how little I spend a month on food. I walk out of the grocery store with sacks of groceries because potatoes, cabbage, onions, papayas, apples, oranges, bananas, and so on are very bulky, giving me a lot for my money, especially relative to meat and refined, packaged products. Inflation costs are always a concern, especially when it comes to food; note that the highest rates of inflation are with beef, chicken, fish, eggs, and dairy.

Some people think that a vegan diet is expensive and that they can't afford it. Well, they can't afford *not* to! A study done at Oxford University and published in *The Lancet Planetary Health* in November 2021 found that "of the seven most sustainable diets, the least costly was the vegan diet."

One of the reasons you save so much money when buying produce is that you are not paying for fancy packaging. You are also not producing so much garbage; this will be one of your contributions to the wellbeing of the planet. Microplastics are now contaminating our beaches and oceans to the extent that they are found in the stomachs of fish and other sea animals, and now even in us humans. Researchers have found microplastic particles in human blood, lungs, and feces and are trying determine what the effects are.[8]

Remember: there's no such thing as throwing "away" your garbage; you're just moving it from one place to another and having someone else deal with it. When you don't buy packaged foods, you are doing your part in protecting the environment from the ravages of industrial society, with its wanton use of plastics to make all this packaging available.

You save even more when you buy fresh produce directly from farms or farmers' markets; it already requires no labor to process, refine, and package natural foods, and you save on transportation cost too. There's also less labor for you. It really doesn't take all that much time to prepare your own foods. You don't need a lot of fancy recipes to make good, nourishing, filling meals—unless you want to. I have written an e-book with over a hundred recipes that meet my CHEF criteria (cheap, healthy, easy, and fat-free). These are recipes that I acquired, simplified by using fewer ingredients, and developed over the years that make fueling your body "a piece of vegan cake." You can find some of these recipes at the back of this book.

Oh yes, here is another advantage that you will enjoy. Clean-up is so much easier and faster with neither grease splatters nor the oily film on the surface of dishes, pots, and pans. A plumber once told me that the main cause of slow, clogged drains is FOG—fat, oil, and grease—so even your kitchen sink drains will cheer! How can you pass up such a deal? You can help yourself to glowing good health, save money, and be an environmentalist at the same time. Indeed, thanks to a report from the Food and Agriculture Organization (FAO) of the United Nations (UN), we now know that animal husbandry is the number-one cause of climate change. It's also a major cause of the loss of rainforests, the lungs of the planet. As the UN warns, "rearing cattle produces more greenhouse gases than driving cars."[9]

A Dual Pandemic: Obesity and Coronavirus

This chapter on nutrition would not be complete without addressing one of the most common plagues of the Western world—obesity—which is now, unfortunately, spreading to other countries as they adopt the Western way of eating. Obesity is actually one of the most common co-morbidities in pandemics such as COVID-19. Thus, what we're seeing is a dual pandemic, with obesity being a symptom of an improper diet in conjunction with a sedentary lifestyle. Actually, we might even say that it's a triple pandemic when we consider what the Western way of eating is doing to our home, planet Earth. She is burning up due primarily to animal husbandry. Stopping animal husbandry would go a long way toward stopping human obesity, stopping pandemics caused by zoonotic viruses, and stopping and reversing our climate crisis.

CHAPTER SIX

STARTING AN EXERCISE PROGRAM

"Okay, okay," you might say. "I'm convinced! I've known for a long time now that I need an exercise program, but I just haven't known how to get started." Maybe you're an ex-exerciser: You tried it and you know what to do; you just haven't been doing it. Or maybe you're a sporadic exerciser: You are gung-ho for a while and then get away from it. Then, when you're ready to get back to it, you have to experience the aches and pains of just getting started all over again. That's when you apply what I suggested in the chapter on changing attitudes.

The Science Is Compelling and Abundant!

There is so much research showing that exercise yields an incredible number of benefits. To understand exactly how the science works, you'd have to take courses in exercise physiology; you'd have to know how to compute a VO^2 max and the maximum heart rate, as well as understand the Krebs cycle, the role of ATP and creatine, and so much more. I took such courses way back in the 1990s. So much more research has been done since then; there is so much more to learn.

One very relevant study published in *Medical News Today* on April 15, 2022, suggested that running just a few times a week can slow the aging process for older adults, promoting mobility and quality of life. In the study, Associate Professor of Kinesiology Duck-chul Lee at Iowa State University followed 55,000 older men and women for fifteen years and found that the runners lowered their risk of heart disease and stroke by 45 percent compared to the non-runners. More surprisingly, those who regularly ran for exercise were better at walking than were those who regularly walked for exercise.[1] And good news for you if you say you don't have time to run: running as little as five to ten minutes a day can add three years to your life expectancy! In fact, Dr. Lee says that more is not necessarily better:

the runners in his study who ran more than an hour a day did not get significantly better results.

Yet another exciting finding from the study was how good exercise is for the brain. Exercise produces a protein in the brain called the brain-derived neurotrophic factor (BDNF), which is important in keeping brain cells alive and producing new ones. In other words, exercise is a way to keep your brain as well as your body fit because it causes new brain cells to grow. In particular, aerobic exercise is what aids the brain in a process called neurogenesis, or the formation of new neurons, which we used to think was not possible. This helps maintain memory and protect against cognitive decline, recall issues, and dementia; it also prevents accelerated aging and a myriad of other physical and mental diseases. Intense and frequent exercise increases circulation, bringing additional oxygen and nutrients to the brain and allowing the brain to produce more BDNF.

Amazingly, we now know that exercise *can* help beat back cancer. Research shows that exercise in skeletal muscles produces proteins called myokines (mentioned in an earlier chapter). Although the study was done on men with prostate cancer, the researchers believe that myokines produced by exercise have similar suppressing effects on other cancers as well. This is true especially for both prostate and breast cancers, which are mostly hormone-driven. In addition to the ability of exercise to decrease both weight and body fat and increase strength, a key takeaway from the study was that there was a significant reduction in the growth of live cancer cells exposed to the after-exercise blood compared to those exposed to the before-exercise blood.[2]

On a personal note, it may well have been my marathon running that was producing myokines and that, together with my diet, helped beat back my stage 4 cancer. Beyond that, I do not doubt that this combination, my continued commitment to exercise and my diet, has benefited me to this very day.

Running and Your Back

Running promotes healthy vertebral disks, the little gelatinous cushions between the vertebrae in the spine. You've probably frequently heard about slipped or ruptured disks. For years, it was thought that the rupturing of the vertebral disks was what caused so many back problems. In actuality, it is usually the weakness of the muscles whose job it is to support those disks and the spine. Running helps strengthen these muscles. Diet plays a role here as well. When capillaries, the tiniest of the blood vessels, get clogged from an animal-based diet, the blood supply is cut off, causing ischemia and therefore pain. This is the same mechanism that causes lower-back pain, chest pain during a heart attack, and strokes.

Really, though, you don't need to go through reams of the latest research; you just need to know that it's there if you ever want to check the details. If you're a rank beginner, however, I don't recommend that you just read a book and go out and run a mile like I did.

Get Checked Out First!

Assuming you are an average or normal weight (they are not the same thing because "average" in the US means overweight) and have not exercised in a while, you should get your healthcare provider's clearance. This is to rule out any hidden problems that could surface as a rude surprise. This is especially true if you're over forty years of age. A physical check-up would also be a good idea if you're young and have never really exercised—if you're the type who escaped physical education classes in high school for any one of a number of possible reasons or if you have always been exercise-phobic.

Once you've been declared basically healthy and cleared to start training, you need to make a plan. Running, power-walking, biking, swimming, and the aerobic exercises researched by Dr. Cooper and discussed earlier are all possibilities. You'll need to decide which you'd like to do. Whatever you end up picking will probably require some equipment. I chose running because it was the easiest and most enjoyable for me, with minimal equipment required as well. When I added biking, swimming, and resistance training, each sport required its own set of equipment, which I will cover later.

A Myth about Running and Your Knees

You may have heard or even believe that running ruins your knees. Even some doctors attribute knee damage to running. Let's debunk this myth right now. As I said, most people and even doctors (with the exception of Dr. Cooper) view impact on the knees as damaging to the cartilage supporting the knees, resulting in osteoarthritis or so-called wear-and-tear arthritis. We now know that impact is actually very beneficial to both bones and cartilage.

For bones, impact causes, via the Piezoelectric Effect, a kind of spark that stimulates the osteoblasts to build more bone. On the other hand, cartilage, or the smooth layer of tissue that cushions the knee and bones of other joints, has a very limited blood supply and so benefits from the Bellows Effect from running. We now know that it's the loading of the body's weight on the meniscus, the specific cartilage on either side of the knee, that, as the body impacts the ground with each stride, squeezes the cartilage like a sponge, expelling metabolic waste and carbon dioxide and drawing in a fresh supply of nutrient- and oxygen-rich blood. As the body springs off the ground for the next stride, there is an unloading. The effect of these loading forces is what explains why, contrary to the myth, most runners have strong, healthy knees.[3]

More evidence of the value of running lies in the results of Stanford University's ten-year-long study following long-term distance runners. (I was actually one of the runners in the study.) They found that these runners had no more osteoarthritis (so-called wear-and-tear erosion of the knee cartilage) or knee replacements than did non-runners.[4]

Another Myth Shattered

It has been generally accepted that cartilage as well as tendons and ligaments turn over much more slowly than do muscles. This has been said to be especially true if an injury or so-called wear-and-tear erosion of cartilage has occurred, which can only be treated with surgery. A 2019 study cast doubt on this tightly held belief. A group of researchers got tissue samples from patients who had just undergone knee surgery and, for the next twenty-four hours, measured cell turnover rates of muscle, tendons, ligaments, and cartilage. They found that fractional protein synthesis rates for the other types of tissue were within the same range as that of muscle cells, 1 to 2 percent per day. They also noted that tissue taken from the back of the knee had slightly lower cell turnover rates than did tissue from the front of the knee, reflecting the fact that we use the muscles on the front of our knees more than those on the back. This is another benefit that exercise provides for our knees.[5]

What You Need to Know about Running

How much do you know about running, if you've decided to try it? If the answer is "not much," then all you need to know for right now is to put one foot in front of the other, lean forward, bring your other foot to catch yourself, and repeat. On the other hand, what there is to know about running can also be so complex that it takes a computer to analyze all that is going on in the body as it moves from point A to point B in a ballistic fashion. Let's start with the basics.

Getting a Running Start!

To get your running start, you'll need a pair of running shorts, a running singlet or t-shirt, and a pair of running shoes. Do not do as I did (dig out an old pair of tennis shoes from the back of my closet); back in 1968, I had no idea there were such things as special running shoes, which were introduced to me one day by my daughter's boyfriend, who ran track in high school. I didn't get my first pair of *running* shoes until 1971—men's, of course, because women's running shoes hadn't even been invented yet. I've just never switched since.

Go to a running-gear store to get the right size and try on several types of running shoes. Many stores will let you do a short run so you can check out the fit of the shoes. A mistake most people make is to buy shoes that are too small, so make sure there's plenty of toe room. Keep in mind that there is no break-in period for running shoes. They need to feel comfortable from the start.

It is important to be comfortable to avoid chafing and possible injuries. Non-running clothes can chafe and bind, so get the high-tech fabrics that wick perspiration away from your body. As you get more into the sport, you can add accessories such as visors, sweat bands, electronic time-pieces to calculate your running pace and splits, and a radio headset or other music-listening device to keep you company in areas where it's safe to run with one.

Take care to get weather-appropriate gear. When it's cooler, you might need tights to keep your legs warm and a warm-up suit for before and after running (for cool-down). You can also buy elastic shoelaces to save you time and effort in putting on and taking off your running shoes. There are new gadgets out on the market all the time, some of which can be very useful. There are heart-rate monitors that range from ear clips to finger sensors to straps around the chest that send telemetry data to a sensor at another location. You'll want to evaluate different accessories on your own. You may find that some of them add to the challenge and enjoyment of your workouts.

Safety First

Always run in well-lit, populated areas and let someone know where, when, and how long you plan to run. Always carry identifying information, including name, address, and an emergency contact name and phone number. Carry a whistle or mace in case you ever need help. Wear bright colors and reflective gear, especially if you run at night, and always run against traffic. For longer runs, in addition to water, carry some nutritional supplements such as vegan fruit bars.

Although I started out running every morning, seven days a week, I don't necessarily advise that. I was lucky in that I adapted quickly to my new routine with no overuse injuries; to be safe, have adequate recovery time and take a day off if you feel you need to.

If you find that you love running and want to make it a part of your lifetime fitness program, I cover it in a lot more detail in chapter 10.

You Don't Need a New Set of Wheels

For the beginning cyclist, things are a bit more complicated. You're fortunate if you already have a bike, even if it's an old "clunker." You don't need a fancy racing machine to start off with. In fact, it's better to wait to make a purchase until you know more about what works best for you. For the time being, almost any bike will do. You might want to get some professional help to properly fit the bike to you, including adjusting the seat and stem heights. I'm afraid no bike is going to be comfortable for the beginning cyclist trying to go for long rides. You will probably hurt in places you never suspected you'd ever hurt! Rest assured that this does pass as your body adapts.

In addition to the basic set of wheels, you will need a safety-approved helmet. It is absolutely crucial that you start out with one since you're more apt to fall early on as you're learning bike-handling skills. Almost every day, I cringe when I see cyclists, moped riders, motorcyclists, and skateboarders riding without a helmet, obviously thinking they are skillful enough to avoid any accident. As a matter of fact, falling is a risk that even cycling experts face, because even if you were perfect, not everybody else is! So play it safe and protect your most valuable asset, your brain.

You will find that things can and do go wrong with your bike, such as flat tires. It will pay dividends to join a bike club and take a course in bicycle mechanics so you can learn how to fix whatever might get broken while you're out on a ride. It also helps to have a bicycle mechanic become your new BFF!

A few simple modifications will turn any old bike into a pseudo racing machine. Add one or two water-bottle cages to the frame to prevent dehydration—a real danger on long rides. You can then unscrew the conventional pedals and replace them with toe-clip or clipless pedals that will add immeasurably to your riding speed, comfort, and safety, but they do require special bike shoes. A racing seat (called a saddle by serious cyclists) won't do much for comfort for a while, but it will be better than the old spring models with which a lot of cruiser bikes are equipped. If your bike has upright handlebars, you can change over to the racer's more aerodynamic drop handlebars.

If you want to go all the way, change the gear clusters so that you can tackle steep hills, switch to racing wheels to decrease your rolling resistance, and add triathlon-style handlebars with elbow pads that put you lower on the bike for a more aerodynamic position. All these modifications can wait, however, until you've had a chance to see how much you enjoy cycling, how competitive you want to be, and how much money you want to put into the sport.

The rest of the cycling equipment is primarily for comfort. Get padded cycling shorts, a cycling jersey, cycling gloves, and cycling shoes to wear. For the uninitiated, a properly outfitted cyclist makes quite a sight. The shorts are skintight, have chamois (or simulated chamois) padding in the crotch, and come midway down the thigh to protect the inner leg from chafing. Luckily, though, cycling shorts seem to be the "in" thing to wear now.

The cycling jersey is also skintight and has funny little pockets around the back. After an hour or so on the bike, you'll learn how convenient these pockets are for storing food, sunblock, and more food. As I've said, your bike should be equipped with water-bottle cages, but for really long rides, you might want to stick an extra water bottle in one of your jersey pockets.

Cycling gloves are fingerless, padded, funny-looking, and colorful. They are fingerless to allow for the unencumbered use of your fingers and padded to help absorb road shock through the handlebars, as well as for when you and the road meet unexpectedly. Cycling shoes come in two versions: touring and racing. Touring shoes look almost like regular shoes, except that the soles are more rigid and there are ridges across the center of the soles to hook into the raised portions of the pedals. They are designed like this so that when you get off the bike, you can walk like a normal person. On the other hand, racing shoes make you walk funny—just the opposite of tip-toeing—due to the cleats that lock into the pedals. These are a little tricky to get used to, but once you've made the conversion, you'll never go back. Herein lies another good reason for always wearing a helmet: novice cyclists (and even some old-timers) sometimes can't get out of the cleats in time and find themselves unceremoniously dumped. Embarrassing but survivable!

The next accessory you'll want is for the bike itself. There are little bags, usually with Velcro straps, that attach to the bike under the saddle. In this little kit, you'll want tools that help you be prepared for flat tires. Add a set of Allen wrenches, a little crescent wrench, a spare tire or tube, a patch kit, some pre-moistened towelettes, and money for a phone call in case all else fails. (You can read more about bicycling in a later chapter.)

Getting Your Feet Wet

If you decide that swimming will be your exercise of choice, all that's required is a bathing suit, goggles, maybe a cap, and of course, enough water. Hopefully, you're lucky enough to have access to either a pool or the ocean. Most serious female swimmers wear both one-piece suits and swim caps for aerodynamics (or hydrodynamics, I should say). Men wear non-boxer swimsuits and swim caps for the same reason. Hair, floppy material, and seams slow you down when seconds count.

Whether you train in the ocean or in a pool, goggles are necessary to protect your eyes from the salt or chlorine, enabling you to see continuously in and out of the water. (If you're swimming in the ocean, as a bonus, goggles will let you appreciate amazing underwater scenery. Some of my most enjoyable ocean swims have been off Waikiki Beach where you can see where the underwater lava flows ran into the ocean years ago.) You also need to see well above the water line on the horizon so that you can navigate accurately. So, get good, well-fitting goggles. There's nothing more miserable than having hard plastic jab you around the eyes, maybe except for trying to see through fogged-up goggles. Find goggles that have an anti-fog coating. My longest swim thus far has been five miles, and while I hurt in a lot of places, thankfully, my head wasn't one of them.

There are miscellaneous training aids that can help allay the boredom of swimming laps. These include hand paddles, pull buoys (foam cylinders that go between your upper inner thighs to raise the lower half of your body and enable you to concentrate on your arm stroke), kick boards (foam boards that you hold onto in order to concentrate on your kick without having to worry about your arm stroke), fins, and a number of resistance gimmicks such as a swimsuit with pockets that make it work like a parachute, or an elastic band tethering you to one end of the pool so that you can swim forever and never have to turn around. (Read more on the benefits of swimming later.)

Keeping Time

There are two recommended items that you might want to have before starting your exercise program, whether it comprises of one sport or multiple different ones. Have a waterproof watch that can measure seconds and a journal (it doesn't have to be fancy). There are a number of exercise logbooks on the market; check any bookstore. Keep track of the type of exercise you do, your heart rate, comments about each day's exercise, and then weekly totals. There should be enough space to record at least a year's worth of data.

This journal will be useful now and in the future. I find it very satisfying to thumb through my exercise journals from years past to see how far I've come.

An optional item that adds considerably to the fun of checking your body's "tachometer" is a heart-rate monitor, which will give you faster and more accurate readings and can even keep you from getting into trouble by letting you know if your heart rate gets too high.

Checking Your Pulse

Now that you've got the basic equipment, you need to assess where you're at. Start with measuring your resting heart rate by feeling your pulse in your wrist or your neck and counting the beats for one minute. Now, nobody I know has the patience to stand there for a whole minute, so just count the beats for ten seconds and multiply that figure by six, or count for six seconds and add a zero to your result. For the greatest accuracy, start counting from zero.

Record this figure in your journal. If you're average, your resting heart rate will be around 72 beats per minute (bpm). Generally speaking, this heart rate will give you an indication of how aerobically fit you are. The lower your number, the greater your fitness. And of course, if your heart rate is higher than the average, just think how much improvement you're going to see!

Next, calculate your maximum heart rate. There are a number of ways to do this, but the simplest is to subtract your age from 220, the theoretical maximum at birth. Let's assume that you are thirty years old; your maximum heart rate would theoretically be 190 bpm. Now, let's calculate your training intensity range. Take 60 percent and 80 percent of 190 (multiply it by 0.6 and 0.8). You now have a range of 114 to 152 bpm. This tells you that if your heart rate is under 114 bpm, your training is probably not intense enough to give you a beneficial cardiovascular effect; conversely, if your heart rate is higher than 152 bpm, it may be too intense and you're courting injury. Your training range lets you design workouts in any sport that will yield aerobic benefits and subsequent improvements in your cardiovascular condition.

In sum, your heart rate gives you the information you'll need to determine how intensely you should train. The next question is for how long. You'll need to get a baseline measurement that will be determined by how fit you are at this moment. Moreover, your fitness level will vary with each sport. You will need to find a course to measure swimming, biking, and running distances accurately. (For example, in my local area, you could use the 25-meter-long pool where I did most of my swim training, the 15-mile route around that area, and the 400-meter track at the university.)

To get your baseline measurements, swim four lengths (100 meters) of a 25-meter pool. Later, when fully recovered, bike a 15-mile loop (or some such distance). Again, when fully recovered and preferably on another day, run a mile (four times around a 400-meter track). Note your time for each test, and you've got some baseline measurements. Also, measure your heart rate at the end of each of the three trials. These should not be done on an all-out basis. Do each test at a pace that is comfortable but not too slow.

It's a little difficult to get your heart rate while doing each of the three sports without a heart-rate monitor, but you can stop and immediately take your pulse manually to give you an idea of the range within which your heart is operating. You will soon get a pretty good feel for your approximate heart rate relative to your level of effort. If you're rolling along very comfortably, barely breathing hard, you can be pretty sure that you're at the lower end of your training range, closer to 60 percent, whereas if you're "dying" and panting, your eyes darting wildly, you are likely operating at or over the upper end. You will soon learn when to push yourself a little harder and when you need to back off on the pace.

Some people have difficulty in finding their heart rate, especially if they are swimming or on a bike. According to one of my physician friends, there is a good correlation between heart rate and breathing rate. What this means is that a high number of breaths per minute compared to your normal breathing rate would indicate a fast heart rate. To find your normal (baseline) breathing rate, count your breaths when you're fully rested. The baseline rate is usually around fourteen breaths per minute. Then check your breathing rate when you're in a rolling-along-comfortably state, which is maybe fifteen or sixteen per minute. This will be within your aerobic envelope, the range within which you want to stay for most of your training. Don't bother with checking out your maximum breathing rate, please. That would get you past your aerobic threshold and into the realm of pain! We don't want you exercising at that level until you are at super-fit levels and going for age-group or elite records.

Planning Your Exercise

You may find that these trial distances are where you need to start and that you can just barely get through the 15-mile bike ride, in which case you can drop the course to 10 or even 5 miles. Or perhaps you find that you are not even breathing hard after the 100-meter swim. In that case, go for 200 or 300 meters. Stop at the point where you are just starting to feel fatigue, measure your heart rate (or breathing rate), and record it.

The same applies to running. It may well be that a mile is a good distance for you to start with. You can then plan gradual distance increases of 5 to 10 percent every other week in all three sports. Look at your personal calendar and decide when to train and how many days a week you can devote to your training. For example, you may be able to swim at noon three days a week—Monday, Wednesday, and Friday. You may want to get your biking in by riding to and from work on Tuesday and Thursday and going for a long ride on Saturday. Running can be done early in the morning, after work, or whenever. Just be sure not to go more than three or four days between workouts for each sport. Conversely, don't schedule workouts too close together without adequate recovery time. Elite athletes can train twice a day, but most of us mere mortals cannot!

You now have enough information to plan several weeks of workouts. For example: Week One might consist of swimming 400 meters on Monday, Wednesday, and Friday; cycling 15 miles on Tuesday and Thursday and 25 miles on Saturday; and running a mile early in the morning Monday through Friday. At the end of the week, review your workouts and make adjustments as necessary.

If you are feeling energetic, strong, and ambitious, you're doing it right. Stay on that schedule for another week (Week Two). By then, you should be ready to increase the distances. Week Three might look like this: swim 440 meters on Monday, Wednesday, and Friday; cycle 16.5 miles on Tuesday and Thursday and 27.5 miles on Saturday; and increase the daily run to 1.1 miles. These gradual increases will allow lots of time for your body to adapt to the new stresses being put on it and will keep you from getting injured.

By Week Four, you'll be able to increase again, assuming that your end-of-week assessments are all still on "go." Don't be afraid to back off if you start to feel soreness or fatigue. On the other hand, though, don't be tempted to jump the schedule by leaps and bounds just because you feel so darned good. That's how many of the "walking wounded" got into trouble!

Speaking of walking, there is a lot of talk about the benefits of walking as a fitness exercise. Naturally, if, for any reason, you are unable to run, walking is an excellent substitute. What you will find, however, is that walking is not nearly as effective or efficient an exercise as is running. It is very difficult to get your heart rate up into your training range, and it takes much more time to cover the same ground. As long as you have not waited too long to start your fitness program, I recommend starting with slow running. You'll be miles ahead (pun intended) if you do! Plus, you'll burn twice as many calories. Scientific research shows that a 160-pound person burns 356 calories for half an hour of running compared to 156 calories for half an hour of walking.[6]

Want a Nice, Flat Stomach?

Consider adding core exercises and weights to your weekly routine. A flat stomach comes about when two conditions exist: strong abdominal muscles to support your internal organs and the absence of excess fat deposits. This is where both daily vigorous exercise and the whole-food, plant-based vegan diet come in. To strengthen your core, there are a number of different exercises: check out the plank, the bridge, and the hanging knee raise. Check with a physical therapist for instructions on how to do these effectively and without injury.

The exercises that do the most for your large muscle groups are: squats, lunges, lat pull-downs, bicep curls, tricep curls, and calf raises. Ideally, we all would have access to a well-equipped gym, but you can do most of these exercises at home with minimal equipment.

HIIT

To get a real workout, try High-Intensity Interval Training (HIIT). It's a protocol whereby you alternate between short periods of intense anaerobic exercise (exercise that doesn't make your body use oxygen) and short recovery periods until near-exhaustion. HIIT training relies on your anaerobic energy, with only short periods of rest. For example, on a stationary bike, you'd turn the resistance up to maximum load, pump for twenty to forty-five seconds, then rest for no more than ten seconds before repeating for another interval. If you go for longer than a minute, your aerobic system kicks in. Thus, you are training your anaerobic system; this is very different from aerobic cardiovascular training. How long a workout lasts depends on your fitness level, but it wouldn't exceed thirty minutes in total. This type of training would be valuable for your running, cycling, and swimming as well, for when you need to expend quick bursts of energy—for example, when trying to beat your previous record's time or making the final push to beat a competitor to the finish line of a race. (However, if you've ever had any heart problems, you'll definitely need to check with your doctor first.)

Overall, I think the ideal exercise program is cross-training—two or three sports plus weights—which will work out all parts of your body and not overstress any one set of muscles. This is why I think doing triathlons has so many benefits. Once your commitment to exercise deepens, you can consider setting up your own home gym with a treadmill, a stationary bike, weights, and even a lap pool. Of course, there are also establishments such as gyms and some YMCAs that provide opportunities for a lifetime of physical fitness. By following a program like the one I just suggested, you'll be developing a triple-sport lifestyle that will make you feel lean, mean, and fantastic—hopefully for the rest of your life. And speaking of the rest of your life . . .

Resistance Training vs. Cardio or Aerobics

There is a lot of evidence that just cardio/aerobic exercise, which is any exercise that uses oxygen and the major muscle groups, might not be enough to prevent sarcopenia, which typically begins around sixty-five to seventy years of age. Sarcopenia—the loss of muscle strength, along with mobility, independence, psychological wellbeing, and quality of life, with aging—has been shown to always occur unless counteracted by resistance (weight) training.[7] Resistance training is an important adjunct to your exercise program, especially as you get older. This can be accomplished using weights, stretch bands, straps, or even your own body weight such as in push-ups, pull-ups, and planks. In order to increase muscle mass, it is necessary to load a muscle with more weight than it has been accustomed to. Therefore, resistance training also needs to be progressive to be effective. When done properly with a frequency of at least once a week, resistance training increases muscle mass as well as stimulates the formation of bone and connective tissue. Indeed, adequate muscle strength and bone density are both extremely important to forestall frailty as we age. As certified personal trainer Scott Hogan has stated: "Load training (a.k.a. resistance training) is the most effective lever for resolving joint pain and building a resilient body. Everything else—stretching, foam rolling, massage, flossing, smashing, taping, cracking, and popping—is secondary."[8] I strongly suggest that you consult a qualified fitness trainer to develop a program specifically for you to keep sarcopenia at bay as you age.

CHAPTER SEVEN

BODY FAT: WHAT YOUR BMI AND SCALES DON'T TELL YOU

Many people seem to be obsessed with their body weight. You hear it in their discussions about food. They talk about all the different diets and methods they've tried—the Paleo diet, the ketogenic or keto diet, portion control, intermittent fasting, weight-loss supplements, calorie counting, exercising to burn off fat, etc. You see the same weight obsession in television commercials, in newspaper and magazine articles and ads, and in supermarkets. The food industry produces advertisements to push food products that do not do what they are supposed to do—that is, nourish our bodies and provide the right amount of fuel needed to give us energy. Regardless of all this attention, a high percentage of our population is either overweight or obese from excessive calories.

Unfortunately, being overweight or obese is linked to a host of debilitating health problems, including heart disease, cancer, stroke, diabetes, and hypertension—most of the major killers of Americans (and Westerners). People in this country spend more than $60 billion a year on trying to lose weight (that figure has gone up from "only" $33 billion a year, which I cited in the first edition of this book).[1] In 2022, nearly 75 percent of us were overweight to some degree, though approximately 50 percent of us were on a diet at one time or another. Indeed, every study shows that we are getting fatter and fatter. And unfortunately, this phenomenon is spreading all over the globe as more countries can afford to switch to a more meat-centered, Western diet, resulting in dual pandemics like I mentioned earlier.

At supermarket checkouts, you see magazine covers splashed with buzzwords like "low-cal," "lite," and "low-fat," along with photographs of skinny models or line drawings of impossibly thin bodies. Most people don't know why they seem to always eat more than they burn off. This is explained by excess fat calories that get converted to body fat, much to the dismay of youngsters, oldsters, men, women—everybody! A lot of the times, even when someone has a normal BMI and doesn't look overweight, they may still be, in reality, "over-fat." (The Body Mass Index does not take into account body-fat percentage.) This is because the body puts the aforementioned excess fat calories not just into more obvious fat deposits, such as in the hips, thighs, and waist, but possibly also in and around the liver, heart, lungs, and intestines. When this happens, fat that is packed around the internal organs puts pressure on the abdominal wall until it bulges out. So, when you look at the profile of a person with a large belly, you are looking at visceral fat, the most dangerous type. The excess fat is also packed between the abdominal wall and skin, making the wearer uncomfortable as well as affecting their self-image. In addition, excess fat is a major cause of sleep apnea, which often reverses when weight is lost.

We have already talked about which foods will provide maximum nourishment to the body and fill the stomach but will not lead to obesity. These are, again, plant foods with the lowest caloric densities. But first, when it comes to losing weight, it's important to understand the concept of body-fat percentage as opposed to body weight. All body weight that is not fat is considered lean body mass—primarily bone, muscle, and water. So, if someone is 15 percent body fat, they are 85 percent lean body mass.

This becomes important when diet and exercise are considered. An extremely low-calorie diet burns off muscle as well as fat, especially if no exercise accompanies the caloric restriction. It will also drastically lower the basal metabolic rate, or the number of calories required to maintain minimal bodily functions. This means that you will put fat on faster if you resume your previous eating habits.

On the other hand, exercise can help retain lean body mass while burning off body fat. It will also help keep the basal metabolic rate up. This is especially important for you in the long run because you don't want your body to learn how to become more efficient in hoarding calories. Take two people, both of whom weigh 150 pounds. One may have a body-fat percentage of only 5 percent, the other 50 percent. The two will look radically different. The person with 5 percent body fat will look very lean with good muscle definition, veins that are obvious through the skin, and contours that suggest a body with very little subcutaneous (under-the-skin) fat. The person with 50 percent body fat, on the other hand, will not look at all lean; their muscles will be hidden under layers of fat, no veins will be obvious through their plump skin, and their contours suggest roundness, obesity, and lack of muscle tone.

These are two extremes. What about people within the range of 20 percent to 40 percent fat? What do they look like? Well, this may surprise you, but a person with 20 percent fat may look just like the person with 40 percent fat. A lot depends on the distribution of that fat. If much of the fat is in the muscles, then the person could look quite lean. You can't tell by appearance alone.

Well, What Should I Weigh?

What about all those weight tables and charts that tell you what you're supposed to weigh? Well, you already know enough about body-fat percentages to see that they (and your bathroom scales) don't really tell you what you want to know. Don't throw them out yet, though. Both are useful in that they give you feedback and a benchmark to start with.

Since it is unlikely that you have ready access to your body-fat measurement, your scale can be the first to tell you that you are gaining weight. Now, since muscle weighs more than fat does, how do you know which you are gaining? Unfortunately, if you are eating the SAD or typical Western diet and leading a sedentary life, you can bet that the weight gain represents excess fat. Your clothes will also be providing clues, as your pants and belts get more and more snug!

On the other hand, if you are not taking in excess calories and are exercising at least five times a week for at least twenty minutes (the minimum required for your body to switch to fat-burning mode), the scale can still show a higher number. This time, however, your clothes will fit more loosely, draping over a much leaner torso. If you want to see what your body would look like with no excess fat, look at the illustrated anatomical chart of the muscles that I've included here. We all have these curves inherently; all you have to do to see them is get rid of the fat that conceals them.

So how do we know how fat we are? There are more than a dozen scientific methods of measuring body composition. Most of them, however, are limited to clinical and research laboratories or the meat industry. Unfortunately, the most accurate methods are the most expensive and the most unavailable.

Currently, the most commonly used estimate is the BMI, which is calculated by dividing your weight in kilograms by your height in meters squared. A normal BMI is considered to be 18–25. Unfortunately, this formula does not consider body-fat percentage, which is important. Alternatively, using your waist measurement as an indicator does help. According to the American Heart Association, waist circumference should measure no more than 35 inches for women and no more than 40 inches for men.

Potassium-40

The most accurate method of measuring body fat to date involves measuring the isotope potassium-40 (^{40}K), although there are a number of other techniques that are now being researched. Unfortunately, the ^{40}K method requires a lead-shielded room and a lot of very expensive equipment to measure minute amounts of gamma radiation.

Electrical Impedance Measurement

Another body-fat-measuring device estimates lean body mass from the body's electrical conductivity. This method is convenient, fast, and not terribly expensive (a test costs around $20 to $50), but unfortunately, it is not very accurate, although it's supposed to be accurate to within ±6 percent. Actually, it seems to do a better job of measuring hydration levels in the body (how thirsty you are). For twelve hours prior to the test, the subject is supposed to fast, especially consuming no alcohol or caffeine, and also abstain from exercise. Within an hour of the test, the subject should not go to the bathroom. For the reading itself, they should lie still for fifteen minutes. (If applicable, they should not be menstruating.) A tiny electrical current is introduced to the body through electrodes placed on the hands and feet. The reading of electrical impedance varies depending on whether this current passes through lean body mass or fat, and an estimate of body composition is derived therefrom. This test has been popular at some running events and triathlons, used by weight-loss-oriented businesses to try to entice new customers.

Near-Infrared Interactance

One of the newer methods is near-infrared interactance (NIR), which uses a tiny light beam that enters the body through a light wand placed on the biceps. The presence of fat changes the spectrum of the light beam. The read-out is quick (about ten seconds) and cheap ($5 to $25), but this test not yet widely available. The accuracy range is supposed to be ±3 percent and is not affected by exercise prior to the reading or hydration levels. There is a major assumption made in the test, however, that cannot be supported: that the fat percentage at the one site of measurement (the biceps) correlates highly with total body fat in all people. This is highly unlikely, as anyone who has done much body-fat testing will tell you.

Calipers

The most convenient and relatively inexpensive but unfortunately least accurate method of assessing body fat is using calipers. These look like large pincers, which is, in fact, an apt description as they pinch the fat under the skin. For accuracy, you would need a well-calibrated, more decently priced set, not the cheap plastic kind usually seen at health fairs. You also need a well-trained person to carry out the test, which involves measuring the thickness of folds of skin at three to nine sites on your body with the calipers, calculating the sum of the measurements, looking up that figure in a chart, and coming up with an estimate of total body-fat percentage. The primary source of inaccuracy stems from the fact that this method measures subcutaneous fat and not any of the "marbling" fat in the muscles. (You've heard of marbled steak as being the most tender. Now you know why!) It also cannot measure any of the fat packed in the abdominal cavity, around the internal organs, producing what we in Hawaii call an *opu nui* or big tummy.

Moreover, people are genetically programmed to store fat in different areas, much to the dismay of women who are prone to "riding-breeches" fat storage, or storing fat on their thighs. The margin of error for skin-fold testing is supposed to be ±3.5–5 percent. Its major value, however, comes from its usefulness as a baseline. Once your initial measurements are obtained, you can then implement changes in your lifestyle and re-measure periodically to see what results you're getting. The best and possibly only solution to excess body fat is to burn up fat stores through exercise and a slight but definite deficit in calories.

Liposuction

There is another solution—liposuction—which will work but which many people feel is rather drastic. Besides its being a costly surgical procedure with attendant risks, the success of liposuction is highly dependent on the skill of the surgeon performing the procedure, which requires the judicious application of large and small cannulas (suction tubes) to suck tunnels through body fat. As such, you can end up with ridges surfacing on your body.

There are other risks to this operation as well, such as asymmetry, which can happen whether you get a liposuction on both sides of the body (a bilateral liposuction) or just one. You could also end up with flabby, loose skin. Most seriously, there have been a number of deaths reported in association with this procedure. Again, you are much better off using a low-fat, low-caloric-density, plant-based diet and a vigorous exercise program.

Hydrostatic Weighing

The last method of body-fat measurement that I will discuss and the so-called gold standard is called hydrostatic weighing, which entails weighing the subject underwater. The theory behind this method is based on Archimedes's Principle, which states that an object immersed in water loses an amount of weight equivalent to the weight of the fluid that is displaced. By submerging an individual on a sling that is attached to an autopsy scale, we can get a weight measurement that determines body density. Using a sophisticated mathematical formula (involving regression equations) and the fact that fat has a density of 0.90 gm/cc and non-fat tissue (lean body mass) a density of 1.10 gm/cc, we then come up with a fairly reliable estimation of body-fat percentage.

The disadvantages to this method are that it's not readily available, it's fairly expensive, and the subject has to be able to expel nearly all of the air from their lungs while underwater. As it is, a lot of people have trouble accomplishing this task, and a very expensive gas-dilution system would be needed to determine accurately the residual lung volume. Additionally, a source error exists in the contents of the gastrointestinal tract; a high-fiber, gas-producing meal can give you an inaccurately high reading.

Getting It Right

An accurate estimate of body-fat percentage can be of crucial importance to an athlete. Rapid weight loss by an already-lean, already-muscular individual can cause severe degradation in athletic performance. More importantly, when muscle is broken down, high levels of urea, ammonia, and purines are released into the blood and can cause kidney damage. In addition, when an adult loses muscle, it is more difficult for them to regain that muscle. In a sedentary individual, this muscle loss might never be recovered and would lead to a higher proportion of fat. This in turn means less calorie-burning tissue, causing the person to gain weight even more easily than before.

This is why I never recommend fasting or extremely low-calorie diets. We want just enough of a caloric deficit to cause the body to burn fat, not muscle. It will burn muscle when it is in starvation mode or even just thinks it is starving—when it isn't getting enough calories. This is one of the most critical points to remember whenever you are tempted to try a calorie-restricted diet, no matter how highly acclaimed it is.

So how much fat should we carry around? You know what starving people look like, so you know that we do need some body fat, which serves several purposes, such as insulation, padding, and energy storage. When you consider, however, that the average thirty-year-old woman is 30 percent fat and the average thirty-year-old man is 10 percent fat, compared to the average female long-distance runner's 6–12 percent and the average male long-distance runner's 4–9 percent, you can guess that the average person has lots of body fat to spare. Note that Ironman triathletes tend to possess a little more body fat than do other runners, probably due to the fact that swimmers in general carry more body fat. In my own experience, training bouts lasting eight to ten hours create an enormous appetite, and I have to eat a lot to sustain the energy levels required to complete that many hours of heavy training. But believe me, I'm not complaining. Eating is the most fun part.

CHAPTER EIGHT

SWIMMING: HOW TO, WHERE TO, AND THE BENEFITS

If you are like me, you learned how to swim many years ago as a child. You may have been taught by your parents or other kids, or as part of a physical education class at school. You probably learned the old-fashioned wheel stroke—that is, arms slicing straight down with no bend to the elbow.

Because I learned to swim when I was three or four, breathing coordination came automatically and was never a problem for me. It's only when I'm coaching new swimmers that the subject of breathing efficiently comes up. There are several basic principles that beginning swimmers need to keep in mind.

Breathing Efficiently

You inhale between arm strokes in the little trough that forms between your head and shoulder. You pivot your head just far enough to the right or left to get your mouth out of the water, then inhale on the sideways upturn of the head and exhale on the downturn as your head goes back into the water. Keep your mouth open and exhale through both nose and mouth. This keeps water out of the nasal and oral passages—well, most of the time anyway. Once in a while, a wave breaks at just the wrong time and you'll gulp a mouthful. Just figure that you're getting a free sip of fluids and keep on going!

Can you imagine the shock I felt when, as I was starting to train for triathlons, somebody told me that I needed to "learn how to swim"? I had been on the swim team in high school and had even been a swim instructor and lifeguard, yet here I was, having to learn a new stroke. It was not quite as bad as learning how to walk all over again, but almost.

Fortunately, colleges, YMCAs, and recreation centers frequently offer swim classes. I signed up for one. On the first day, we saw a film demonstrating the proper arm stroke, which entails bending the elbow at a 90-degree angle and moving the arm in a slightly S-shaped motion. The theory goes that you need to keep "new" water moving. With the old straight-through wheel stroke, you are just moving the same water and thus are not moving ahead as fast as when you are sculling from side to side and grabbing new water continuously, much like how a propeller moves through the air. On the second day of the course, we were videotaped while swimming and shown what we were doing normally. Then we were taught the proper stroke and videotaped again. What a difference! Although the new technique felt very awkward at first, it was not long before there was no question in my mind that this was a much better way to swim. I was also shocked to see in the videotape how low in the water my legs dragged, but once I did, it was no trouble to change my kick and tilt my pelvis so as to keep my legs and feet close to the surface. My swim times began to improve immediately. So, if you are one of the old-school (or no-school) swimmers, get yourself to a good swim coach and learn the most efficient stroke. It'll pay dividends right away.

Another suggested change to my swimming technique came from the "Swim Doctor" himself, Jan Prins, PhD, a well-known and respected swim coach, formerly at the University of Hawaii. His research covers swimming-stroke mechanics, complete with before and after underwater videos. He was the one who taught me bilateral breathing—to alternate sides when I breathe with each stroke—another new trick that was awkward at first but that, as I adapted, I realized provides great advantage, especially in open-ocean triathlon swimming wherein there are no black lines like at the bottom of a pool to follow. In this case, you need to know how to navigate so as to make a beeline to any turns and autocorrect as you go along. Once, during the swim portion of the New Zealand Ironman, a swimmer about six feet away on my right started heading my way and was about to run into me. When I reached out and tapped him on the shoulder, he looked so startled and immediately course-corrected. If he'd been doing bilateral breathing, this never would have happened.

If you're a more recent vintage swimmer, you are already ahead of the game and will need to just get back into a good training program. In this sport, as in most others, the social aspects can be very important. I've always found training in a group with a good coach fun!

Even Adults Need Toys

In the chapter on starting an exercise program, I covered the basic equipment, required and optional, for swim training. I recommended getting "toys," such as pull buoys, kick boards, fins, and hand paddles, that can help relieve the boredom of swimming laps in a pool, which is where most people have to train, and that can moreover give you a more efficient workout.

Swimming in the ocean is nice, but most people do not have access to open waters, and it is almost impossible to measure and time your laps. In any sport, the importance of feedback cannot be overestimated; swimming is no exception. Positive reinforcement gives you joy and pride in your progress, and if you can't measure your progress, you're at sea, literally and figuratively.

There is one disadvantage, though, in doing all your training in a pool. Every 25 or 50 meters or yards (the length of the pool), your back muscles get a rest as you scrunch up to push off against the wall. Then, when you have to do a long swim in a triathlon, your back muscles are unaccustomed to having to hold the same position for a half-mile, a mile, or the standard 2.4 miles in an Ironman. I mentioned earlier that you need to train yourself to be able to navigate in open-ocean swimming because there are no black lines at the bottom of the ocean. Not too many triathlons with open-ocean swims have underwater course markers, although I've actually seen them once (the Wailea Triathlon on Maui had a line on the ocean floor that traversed the entire swim course).

Barring that, though, it's amazing how many people unwittingly add a lot of distance to their swim by heading off in a different direction from that in which they intend to go. While you can just lift your head to see where you're going, this ruins your form and speed. You can't always depend on others for navigation either. In addition to cases of individual deviation like the one that I mentioned during the New Zealand Ironman, I've seen whole packs of swimmers go off course during a race.

You may notice that while swimming, if you have to cough, you'll have a tendency to do it underwater rather than while your face is out of the water, grabbing a breath of air. Your lungs always have some residual air. You cannot exhale all the air from them, even if it feels like you can. If, however, you cough underwater, you are tapping into that residual air, which throws off your breathing rhythm and makes you feel as if you need to gasp for air. You may have to break the nice, smooth pattern of your breathing to get more air sooner. This is better than going into oxygen debt. Try to maximize the amount of oxygen going to your muscles by keeping your lungs as full as possible.

When you're doing ocean swimming in a triathlon, it's very important to orient yourself at the beginning of the swim leg. Being off just a few degrees can add considerably to your fatigue and your time. Pick a tree, a building, or anything that you can see while you're in the water to aim for. Once in a while, during a rough ocean swim, the waves can be high enough to make it difficult to see your landmark. That's when you check ahead to see where the other swimmers are, keeping in mind that they may be having trouble too. In this case, go with the majority until you have more evidence.

Another tip to keep in mind when you're doing ocean-swim legs in events that have course turns marked by buoys: sight the buoys as soon as you can, aim directly for them, and cut the corners so close that you actually brush the buoys. Of course, you may find that a lot of other competitors have the same idea. Charge on ahead and get through the choke point as quickly as possible.

A skill that will also help you in navigation, balance your upper-body muscular development, and distribute your fatigue is bilateral breathing, which I mentioned earlier. Of course, you do need to keep your eyes open. Normally, I would not have thought this an obvious thing to mention until one day when I was talking to my favorite training partner, Kate. After Kate's first 2.4-mile, Ironman-distance ocean swim off Waikiki, I remarked on the beauty of the black lava flows in the ocean, alternating through the white sands off Diamond Head, and of all the beautiful fish we'd passed. She revealed for the first time her fear of the ocean. She'd had to swim almost the entire 2.4 miles with her eyes squeezed shut!

Kate is by no means unique. There are a fair number of brave souls who have to conquer agoraphobia (a fear of wide-open spaces), a fear of sharks, plus a normal, healthy fear of the hazards of open-water swimming. Boats and other over-water crafts have trouble seeing swimmers in the ocean, and moreover are not used to having to look for them.

Swimming Safely

For this reason, always wear a brightly colored swim cap and keep a constant watch for all types of watercrafts. Always swim with a buddy, although unfortunately, nothing precludes both of you from getting run over, as accidents involving multiple swimmers have happened. Safety is another good reason to practice bilateral breathing as it enables you to keep an eye on everything around you. Just don't forget to keep casting your eyes about and even behind you as boats and other watercrafts can quickly overtake you.

Avoiding Boredom

One aspect of pool training we all have to deal with is the boredom associated with just going back and forth. As I'm preparing for a training session in a pool, this thought comes up frequently. There have been a couple of times, such as after a surgery (one of several), when I went to the pool but was unable to swim, not being allowed to by my doctor until my stitches were taken out. I would sit there watching other people go from one end of the pool to the other, then back again, thinking how boring that must be.

Then, one day, I was back in the pool after a forced lay-off. As I started concentrating on the many aspects of my stroke and responding to my swim coach's frequent exhortations to get my elbows higher, all of a sudden, I realized that an hour and a half had passed in a flash. I came to understand that what the out-of-the-water observer sees bears no resemblance to what is actually going on under the surface!

A Word about Wetsuits

Swimmers have discovered that the higher in the water they can swim, the less the frontal resistance. The less the frontal resistance, the faster they go. A wetsuit is buoyant and therefore keeps you higher in the water. That's why you will see lots of swimmers wearing wetsuits in both warm, tropical waters and the chilly waters of northern climes. A wetsuit will also prevent hypothermia, the lowering of your body temperature, so it is at times also a piece of safety equipment. All in all, it is a definite asset to the swimmer's closet.

Even if you never intend to become a triathlete, swimming is one of the best forms of exercise: it is excellent training for your cardiovascular system, is gentle on your joints, and stretches you out. If you have a lot of weight to lose, it may be one of the only aerobic exercises you can do until you get your weight down. It's a good idea to learn to enjoy it and to do it as close to daily as possible. Science shows that swimming is even good for your bones, as it increases bone turnover, which is what keeps bones strong and more resistant to fracture.[1] Swimming is a sport you can practice for the rest of your life, long after you might have to give up cycling and running.

CHAPTER NINE

CYCLING: GETTING MECHANICAL

One of the things that make the cycling leg of a triathlon unique is that it is the only leg in which failure can be attributed to a piece of equipment. After all, you can run barefoot if you lose your shoes, and you can swim without goggles if you lose them or if a strap breaks, but there's no way you can do the cycling leg without a functioning bicycle.

For the mechanically challenged, getting on an equal footing with your bicycle can be pretty intimidating. I've seen young, macho men look at a derailleur (gear shifter) and recoil in horror. On the other hand, I've seen fashion-plate women with long, red fingernails dig right in with wrenches and come out with the greasiest, dirtiest hands. The point is: anybody can learn the basics of bicycle mechanics.

The most fun way to learn how your bike operates is to sign up for a course such as Smart Cycling.[1] Besides learning about bike operation, you'll find out what to look for when buying a bike and how to fit it to your body; also covered are topics such as simple and complex repair and maintenance, safety maneuvers, riding in traffic, bike touring, and much more. In many parts of the country, you can find courses that teach people how to ride bicycles for health, recreation, and transportation.

Upon completion of such a course, you will have been transformed into a confident, competent cyclist. You will know your rights on the road and how to merge safely with automobile traffic. You will have learned to watch a car's front wheels to know which way and when it's going to turn. You will be familiar with bailout maneuvers and panic stops, and if all else fails, you will at least know how to fall properly.

Caution: Be Careful!

Now, if I've made cycling sound a little dangerous, know that it is. I've been hit on the road twice, as I'll talk about later. There's no question that there's a great deal of risk involved in placing yourself on the road, where the automobile has been king for so long. Though there are now dedicated bike lanes in some cities, you still have to be very weary of cars that do not look for you or treat you as if you were invisible, especially at intersections. Many motorists tend to view cyclists as petty annoyances, who belong on the sidewalk or the playground and who have no right to impede the automobiles barreling down the road at breakneck speed. There are even aggressive motorists who, when screaming insults at you and narrowly missing you don't seem adequate, will literally try to run you off the road. This is a problem national and local cycling organizations are grappling with through educational and legislative efforts. Unfortunately, both approaches are slow and run into many obstacles.

It is important to teach proper cycling skills to kids from the time when they get their first bikes. Unfortunately, kids are now taught haphazardly, sometimes erroneously, and that is why you will even see some ride against traffic. But trying to get cycling into the school curriculum, which many consider already overfull, is difficult. Most people don't realize that through cycling, kids can learn a lot about the basic laws of physics, courtesy, physical fitness, nutrition, and independence as well as gain a mode of transportation that frees them from the tyranny of automobiles for the rest of their lives. Idealistic? Perhaps. But when you consider our society's present dependence on fossil fuels, which pollute the very air we breathe, and the fact that more and more kids are growing up obese and physically unfit, you can see how the lowly bicycle can transform our lives in some very positive ways.

In Hawaii, traffic congestion has reached near-gridlock dimensions. People have to get up earlier and earlier to get to their jobs on time. They joke about paving the island over with freeways and parking lots, which is hardly a joke anymore. Lifestyles in "Paradise" have been modified to the point where most people would be hard-pressed to see any difference between living in Honolulu and living in Los Angeles—except that Los Angeles has more bike paths! If more people would get on their bikes to ride to and from work or school, they could relieve some of the congestion on the roads and reduce the need for parking lots. They would also save lots of money, get their exercise/training in during the time that they'd ordinarily spend sitting in a traffic jam, and arrive at work or school feeling wonderfully invigorated instead of irritable.

Don't Sweat the Sweat!

"Ride my bike to work or school?" I hear you asking incredulously. "I might get a little sweaty," you say. "Just where do I shower?" you want to know. That's not a problem! If you start out with clean clothes and you already eat a non-animal-food diet, your sweat doesn't smell bad. It's the breakdown of animal products that causes the typical meat-eater's characteristic body odor. And besides, you're using a different set of sweat glands when you're exercising.

We humans have two different kinds of perspiration glands. One set of glands, the eccrine, secretes moisture to cool the body and carry off some of the waste products of the metabolism. Fresh sweat of exertion has very little odor. It is only after bacterial decay sets in, hours later, that you get the typical locker-room smell, and this is generally from clothes that have not been laundered soon enough. The second set of sweat glands is the apocrine, which does not generally operate when we exercise. It's the apocrine glands that start functioning when we reach adolescence and give off pheromones, that musky scent evolutionarily used for mate calling that some of us try so hard to mask with deodorants and dangerous aluminum-based antiperspirants.

After your commute to work or school, you can always go to the restroom and take a sponge bath. A quick change of clothes, a comb through your hair, a little make-up if you're a woman (although you certainly won't need to add that nice, healthy-looking glow to your complexion since you'll already have it), and you can bounce into the office or classroom feeling enthusiastic and wonderful! If you're a little fearful about appearing "odd," try to talk some of your work or school pals into riding with you. Then cycling becomes absolutely fun, and the bonding that occurs while riding with others gives you a head start on all your relationships with your colleagues or peers. There are all kinds of benefits to be realized.

Beating Gridlock Traffic

Depending on how far from work or school you live, you may get all your training in at no extra cost in time spent. You may even reach your destination faster than you would by driving! If you get really enthusiastic about cycling, you might be out on the road on Saturdays and Sundays too. If that's the case, you'll have no trouble getting in lots of training miles. If you're like most people, however, it's a little more difficult to get those miles up to where you want them. Even if you ride to and from work or school every weekday, it still might not be enough to achieve the total weekly mileage you need for triathlon training. That's when long weekend rides are a must. Try to find a cycling club with a group of riders who are at or a little above your competitive level. Not only will you get some good training but you will also improve rapidly and be safer, riding as part of a group.

There are also different types of rides. All rides can be broken down into two basic categories: endurance training and interval training. Endurance training works out your legs, heart, lungs, and *okole* (as we in Hawaii say "rear end") to be able to hang in there for the long haul. A ride in this category may be 25 miles for a beginner, but for the old-timer, it could be 200 miles, also called a double century!

Don't make the mistake that I made in my early days of training. I thought that cycling was easy, that it was just a matter of getting on the bike and pedaling; it seemed to me like I could go on that way forever. I certainly found out differently when, as I mentioned earlier, I got off my bike at the end of the cycling leg of my first triathlon and my rubbery legs could hardly support my body, much less let me run.

A weekly long-distance ride will probably fulfill your endurance-training requirement. To take care of interval training, you need to set up a program wherein you get out on a road with little to no traffic once or twice a week and do a workout along a pre-measured course, constantly alternating between hard cycling and recovery. Maybe add a little HIIT training as we discussed earlier. Your heart rate will tell you how hard and for how long you can go.

Checking the Heart Rate

Start out by going very hard for a set period of time, measured by a watch or a cycle speedometer. As your heart rate approaches 90 percent of your maximum, back off until your heart rate drops down to 60–70 percent.

Then repeat the process three or four times. I can assure you that you'll have an excellent workout.

If you don't have a heart-rate monitor, trying to measure your heart rate the old-fashioned way will be more difficult. But you'll soon get the hang of it, as your pounding heart will let you know it is being pushed. When you can no longer feel that pounding and your breathing starts to approach normal, you can guess that it's time to go again. If this doesn't sound like a lot of fun, it's probably because it isn't. I also have the most trouble with this part of my training program. Here is another case in which working with a group helps provide motivation.

In an earlier chapter, we've already covered a little about how to modify your old clunker into a racing machine and why cyclists wear what they wear. Cycling technology is such that there is always new equipment out on the market. You can easily find bike houses' websites and get on their mailing lists so you can be notified of the latest products. It's also a good idea to subscribe to at least one cycling magazine to get periodic updates and receive regular doses of motivation.

Cycling is a sport that relies on a piece of mechanical equipment, which can, by its very nature, fail on occasion, often at the worst possible moments. View each of these mechanical failures as an opportunity to learn and rehearse what you'd do in a race. If your buddy is an old hand at fixing flat tires and you're terrified by the mere thought of it, offer to change their flat. This way, you get real-life practice under supervision. As you get that rear wheel through the maze that is the chain, cogs, and derailleur, you'll be unbelievably proud of yourself. What's more is that you'll have lost your fear of getting a flat under extreme pressure. You'll know that you can handle it.

There are lots of other things that can go wrong. As you pile up mileage on the bike, you'll be exposed to them first- or second-hand. Never miss an opportunity to stick your nose into any mechanical crisis. Even if you've studied the problem and handled it in the past, you can probably still benefit from a review and help teach others at the same time. You'll feel so much more comfortable on the bike if you know you can handle the common malfunctions that will catch up with you sooner or later.

On another note, check out spin classes, which are offered at some gyms and which can give you a real workout. I've always finished a spin class totally wiped out, with puddles of sweat on the floor! I attribute my winning first overall in the Las Vegas Senior Olympics to my spin-class training. Joining one of these classes is an excellent way to train safely and effectively. Besides, you meet the nicest people there!

CHAPTER TEN

Running: Getting Fast and Staying Uninjured

I started running back in the days when there was not a great deal published about the sport. You may recall my story of my fateful encounter with Dr. Kenneth Cooper's strangely titled book *Aerobics* at a newsstand in July 1968.[1] You may also recall how I was intrigued by this new word (which Dr. Cooper had just coined), bought the book, and got so engrossed in it that I read it in one sitting (mainly because I skipped over most of the actual data and tables presented from his extensive research). I was drawn to Dr. Cooper's concept of aerobic exercise and how it affects every body part and bodily system, quite literally from head to toe, especially since at the grand old age of thirty-three, I did not have the faintest idea of just how critical both diet and exercise were. I was also plagued with a horrible assortment of maladies, including two ruptured disks, insomnia, constipation, borderline–high blood pressure, and a tendency to gain excess weight. With each chapter that I read, I found a possible solution to a health problem of mine. I was anxious to try exercise.

The easiest of all the exercises described in the book was running. It was also the most convenient, effective, and efficient. It required no special equipment; it could be done alone, at any time and in any place. It seemed ideal for me. I went out for my first run (in my old tennis shoes yet!) the next morning and have been hooked ever since. On my journey, I've sought out and read almost everything I could get my hands on that dealt with running. I've always found the subject fascinating, and it seems that research keeps coming out that supports lifelong running or exercise in general.

Learning nearly everything the hard way, I have also experienced seemingly every injury the body can sustain. What can put you at high risk of injury is doing too much, too soon. How much is too much? Your body will let you know. For beginning runners, there are all sorts of bodily signals that something new requires some adapting to, such as foot pains, chest tightness, shin splints, sore quadriceps (thigh muscles), and so on. At that point, you just back off a little. You don't have to stop—just slow down. You may even need to walk for a while, but do keep moving. Gradually increase the time or distance as your body and schedule allow. Keep track of your time and the distance covered and be consistent in your program.

For starters, schedule maybe just ten minutes for a jog, preferably first thing in the morning. Plan on making it a new habit and do it every morning. If you have to skip one, get right back to it the next day. I suggest you do it in the morning because that's when your energy levels will be charged up, and you can get your workout for the day done and over with. Then, emergencies, minor crises, and especially temptation will not call a halt to your program.

Now, you will not necessarily be running for the full ten minutes. You will run according to your fitness level and walk to round out the time. A great rule to remember is: run until it hurts; walk until it doesn't. If you can run for only two minutes or less for your first time out, that's okay. Walk for the rest of the time. The next day, aim for a little more than two minutes. If your body parts are hurting, stop for the day and let your body recover. If nothing is complaining, increase your running time by a few more minutes. Or, if you go around the block the first time, go for two blocks the next time.

If you're just starting an exercise program, set your goal for twenty-one days. During the first twenty-one days, let nothing interfere with your scheduled workout time, which will preferably be first thing in the morning because of the advantages listed above. Why twenty-one days? Some research shows that it takes around that long to establish a new habit (although the exact figure varies, and it also depends on the positive or negative reinforcement you're getting). Again, working out first thing in the morning is a fantastic way to start your day as well as to ensure your long-term success. Studies show that the most successful exercisers are morning exercisers as early workouts also fit with our diurnal or circadian cycles.[2]

The two main points that you must remember are: be consistent and increase slowly. If you do both, your body will complain a little bit but not too much. If you're an old hand at running, both principles still apply. I believe that everybody needs daily exercise, so join the daily-running club, just alternate between hard or long runs and easier or shorter ones. That's why keeping a log is so important. You need to monitor the intensity and distance of each run so that you don't overdo it yet still keep improving.

Make It Hurt Just a Little **but** *Not Too Much!*

If your body is always totally comfortable, it could be because you're not increasing the stress on it. If you're not increasing the stress on your body, you're not getting stronger or faster. So a little discomfort is a good sign. Remember: run until it hurts; walk until it doesn't. You also need to ensure that you don't overdo it and get yourself injured. A pretty safe rule is not increasing your distance by more than 10 percent a week or month once you get to a mile or two a day.

Again, how much is "too much"? Other than the bodily signals mentioned earlier, your log or journal will offer an excellent way to keep track of your training. Because I train in not only running but also biking and swimming, I sometimes feel that my training is much like juggling—I barely get one ball into the air and another is about to fall. I finish a bike ride and a swim workout is almost overdue. The only way that I know where I stand in each sport is by keeping a running tally in my log.

Another measure that I find valuable is my weekly total workout hours. By monitoring this number, I can pick up trends in my training time (especially downward trends, which are unfortunately sometimes the case). By keeping my weekly totals relatively constant, I know that the demands I'm putting on my body are within range.

The equipment you would need for running was touched upon in the chapter on starting an exercise program. The main points to remember are that you need good shoes (well-fitting, with not too many miles on them), comfortable clothing (nothing that chafes or binds), and a source of water. Running can cause you to sweat a great deal, and it may take only a very small percentage of fluid loss to cause real dehydration-induced problems, including not only loss of performance but also disorientation, possible permanent kidney damage, and lots of things you don't ever want to have happen to you.

That's why you need to stay hydrated, but how do you know much to drink? Remember this tip: it takes about eight or nine swallows to get enough fluid into the stomach to activate the pylorus, the valve that opens to let stomach contents into the small intestine, where the water starts getting absorbed into the blood stream. Here's another test: your urine should be clear. If it's not, you need to drink more water. Remember the three Cs: clear (almost), colorless (light yellow), and copious (lots of it)!

If you're an average adult, you probably have a fairly decent running form. Most people's feet track fairly straight along the line in which they're moving. Their arms hang loosely from their shoulders—with elbows bent at about a 90-degree angle—and swing easily back and forth in rhythm with their legs. And most people are fairly relaxed in their lower arms, neck, and head. If, however, you're not average, you may have some type of running-form abnormality. It's always a good idea to find a running coach and have your running stride analyzed. (The real pros even have their forms analyzed by computer.)

A good coach can quickly tell you if, for example, your head is cocked to one side, you are carrying your arms too high, or you are throwing your legs out to the side as you run. If you have an abnormality, it may well be that you are compensating for some variation in your body's center of gravity, which is changing constantly as you run. If this is the case, there will be no need to change your running form. Just have someone look at you from time to time to be sure that no odd little quirks creep in that could cause you injury or slow you down unnecessarily.

Running Is Not Boring!

One of the most frequently asked questions a runner gets asked is, "Don't you find running boring?" My answer to that question is, "Not even close." Besides thinking about the training I'm doing, my mind tends to cover a myriad of things, and I sometimes find myself hardly aware that any time has passed. Put me with a group of people, and we are laughing, joking, solving our problems, and feeling wonderfully close as a result. Or, although not as likely, we might just run together in silence, sharing in the feeling of our bodies hard at work.

As your running mileage increases, you will find that your mind either associates or dissociates. This means simply that mentally, you either stay tuned in to your running or go off somewhere else. I find that I do both. I usually start a run associating. I think about a slow, gentle warm-up as I gradually increase my heart rate and get cold, tight muscles to loosen and warm to the task. Then I slowly quicken my pace but never to a point where I'm uncomfortable.

After a while, my mind starts to wander. If I'm bothered by a problem, it'll start gnawing at me, and very often, a solution presents itself. A run is also a wonderfully creative time for me. Ideas keep popping up in my head, sometimes so many that I really get excited. In fact, many of the ideas for this book were created on the run, so to speak. Usually, however, by the time I get home, some of those spontaneous ideas have evaporated. There's nothing so fragile and fleeting as ideas, and if you don't capture them right away, they might be gone forever. You can use your smart phone to make notes of good ideas that occur on a run.

There is a scientific basis for the mental stimulation and the burst of creativity and problem-solving inspiration produced by exercise. When we are engaged in aerobic exercise, the brain is getting extra oxygen, leading to not only a short-term stimulating effect on thought processes but also a long-term effect in the form of increased blood circulation. The brain develops larger, cleaner arteries and forms more capillaries. Remember that exercise produces BDNFs, or brain-derived neurotrophic factors. As a result, aerobically fit people think more clearly and creatively and even lower their risk of dementia.

Running Is Actually Good for Your Knees

Another question frequently asked of runners, which was touched on earlier, has to do with whether running is really bad for the knees. People incorrectly think that running wears out the meniscus, a piece of cartilage on each side of the knee joint, leading to "wear-and-tear" arthritis. In actuality, damage to and pain in the knee's meniscus can occur when a bit of foreign protein gets into the joint and triggers an autoimmune response that causes the body to attack its own cartilage.[3] This problem is most often caused by animal protein in the diet, not by running.

You may recall from an earlier chapter that running actually benefits the knee's meniscus. The compression during the weight-bearing stage squeezes the blood out of tiny capillaries; then, when you're airborne, the blood rushes back in, pushed by the increased blood pressure from running.[4] A study that observed nearly five hundred runners over a period of eight years found that they developed only a fifth as many knee and leg problems as did non-runners. Women reaped the most benefits, with almost 90 percent fewer knee problems compared to their non-running counterparts.[5]

The Amazing Tarahumara Runners

Have you ever heard of the Tarahumara Indians in Copper Canyons, Mexico? A people whose diet mainly consists of the "Three Sisters" of indigenous agriculture (corn, squash, and beans), they are known to run races of up to forty-eight, even seventy-two hours, carrying around their waists little bags of ground corn—at an altitude of 7,200 feet! I wanted to see this feat for myself and possibly run a few miles with the Tarahumara runners.

This, however, was no easy task. The Tarahumara, 60,000 in number, live in Copper Canyons or Barrancas de Cupre, an isolated area in northern Mexico. To get there, we traveled by bus to El Fuerte, then boarded the El Chihuahua Pacifico train, known colloquially as El Chepe. The train climbed from near sea level to almost 8,000 feet, crossing thirty-nine bridges and going through eighty-eight tunnels, with switchbacks so extreme that we could see ourselves coming and going!

The next morning, I was all set to meet some of the Tarahumara runners near the hotel where we stayed. There they were, running back and forth, laughing and obviously having fun. I noticed none were wearing running shoes. Their feet were shod in soles cut out of old tires and fastened with sisal rope. I jumped in and, laughing too, ran up and down the short course. Thinking what a fantastic running experience I was having and that I had to get a photograph, I realized, to my dismay, that I'd forgotten my camera!

The Kenyan and Ethiopian Runners

Having run many marathons, I've noticed that when Kenyan runners were entered, they usually won or took most of the top places. The same was true of Ethiopian runners. I checked out their diets. It turns out that Kenyans and Ethiopians eat almost entirely plant-based foods, with vegetables coming straight from the garden. They eat approximately 77 percent carbohydrate, 10 percent protein, and 13 percent fat—about the same proportions that I've been following for over forty years now.[6]

Running for Us Mere Mortals

Have you ever heard of the talk test? Most of the time, your running speed should be at an aerobic level, meaning that you are getting enough oxygen. Simply put, you should run at a speed that is slow enough that you have enough breath to carry on a conversation. If you're huffing and puffing while trying to talk, you are on the edge of anaerobic running and need to slow down.

Running training in general should be aerobic. It's only when you have an adequate mileage base—say, 30–40 miles per week—that you can begin to think about anaerobic training or HIIT, discussed earlier, by adding intervals to your workouts at the track, for example. When you get to this stage in your running training, join a running group with a coach. You'll find that almost any area has some good running coaches associated with high schools, colleges, or community running clubs.

Once you join a group, your running will improve dramatically. You will find, first of all, that your enjoyment of the sport increases, which alone tends to boost your training. But more important is the discipline that group sessions encourage. The structure imposed by a coach and a regularly scheduled meeting time is invaluable in keeping you motivated.

Coaches are also important sources of information. As you increase your running distance and intensity, you may be faced with various aches and pains. It's important to know when such messages from your body constitute a signal to back off in order to prevent injury. It's also interesting to note that we can tell ourselves something, but it never seems to have as much credibility as when we hear it from someone else, especially someone with authority. So get a coach!

Running as an exercise or sport seems to just grab some people, while for others, it's a crushing bore. If you're like me and you love it, the need to increase the distance of your longest run seems almost insatiable. When you have completed your first 10K run, you think about a 15K. Then you start to think about marathons and ultra-marathons. You may even start contemplating running marathons in different locales, as I have done in Moscow, New York City, Boston, and Jacksonville (Florida), to name a few cities. Marathons are held literally all over the world, even in Antarctica!

For some, these extremely long races present a challenge that is appealing and exciting. As they cross the finish line of their first marathon, they usually think one of two thoughts. They may think, *There, I did it, and I'm done!* Or they may think, *Wow, if only I'd trained a little harder, I could have knocked ten minutes off my time!* As you can guess, I fell into the latter category, and I really did start knocking minutes off my time when I changed my diet. At the next marathon that I ran, just four months after my cancer diagnosis and three months after surgery, I beat my own previous best time by seventeen minutes.

Programming the Mind

One of the comments that I hear the most from people is that they cannot imagine running a marathon as the third event of the Ironman. As a matter of fact, when I finished my first 100-mile bike ride, with the way I was hurting, I could not even conceive of *beginning* a marathon. The major difference between that first 100-mile bike ride and my first Ironman was in my mental programming, or goal setting. When I climbed onto the bike the morning of my first 100-miler, I knew that all I had to do was those 100 miles. That was why I didn't collapse at 50 miles, 80 miles, or any distance less than 100 miles. On the other hand, the morning of my first Ironman, I programmed my mind to prepare for a 2.4-mile swim, a 112-mile bike ride, and then a 26.2-mile run. Now, I *did* have to have done the physical conditioning to enable my body to support my mind in accomplishing that goal. I knew that despite feeling intense fatigue at the 80-mile mark of the bike ride, I still had a marathon to go. I did not give my mind any choice in the matter.

The goal was set. My body had been sufficiently trained to support that goal, and the rest, as they say, was history. As a matter of fact, I have never *not* finished a race. I may have given up on setting any records for a given race, but I've found that I can always dig a little deeper. To me, finishing a race has always been more important than anything else, and the positive reinforcement from finishing has just kept that principle going.

I recall that at the 22-mile mark of my first marathon, I decided that I would never again put myself in a position of such extreme discomfort. About that time, a nice, good-looking young man came up and started running with me. He, too, was "dying." Just then, I got an idea. I knew that if we could dissociate for just a bit, we could probably get through that marathon. So, I asked him if he wanted to try an experiment to help get us through. He, of course, agreed. I told him to visualize the most exciting erotic experience he'd ever had or would like to have.

He looked surprised, smiled, and said, "Okay, I got one!" He shared his, and I shared mine, and the next thing I knew, the finish line was in sight and we sprinted for it! That experience taught me a bunch. At about the same point in the marathon of my first Ironman, I was feeling totally depleted and wondering how I was ever going to finish when I recalled my first-ever marathon. I then dropped back to the person behind me, who turned out to be Duke, a friend.

Duke was absolutely miserable. His running shoes had been lost at the transition from his bike, and he'd been offered someone else's shoes in a desperate, last-ditch effort to save the race. Duke had not only trained hard for a year for this event, he'd also traveled all the way from Saudi Arabia, where he was stationed in the Army, just to compete. The shoes were way too small, and Duke was bloodied and almost beaten. We started dissociating, and of course, you know the rest. There never was a more welcome sight than the Ironman finish line for both of us that day!

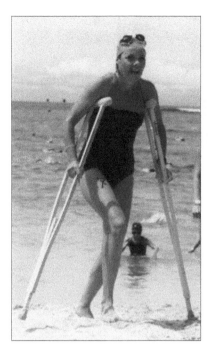

Coming up on the finish line of the Waikiki Roughwater Swim two weeks after a pelvic fracture, using crutches to get into and then out of the water. I could not do any weight-bearing activity while recovering from being hit by a truck on a training bike ride. My first Ironman was seven weeks later, for which I was told I'd never heal in time. I proved that prediction wrong.
September 3, 1984.

Completing the Windward Half Marathon with braces, three days after just having been diagnosed with hot spots in both legs.
May 8, 1984.

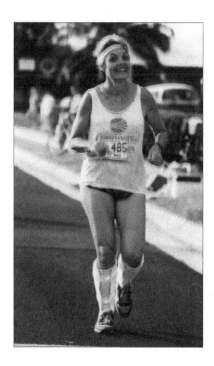

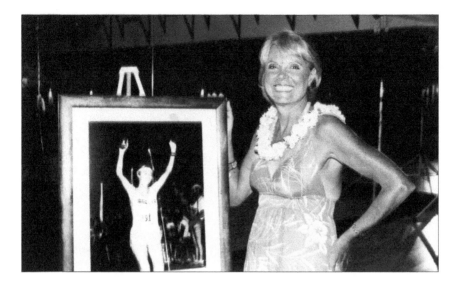

Being inducted into the Gold's Gym Hall of Fame.
October 1997.

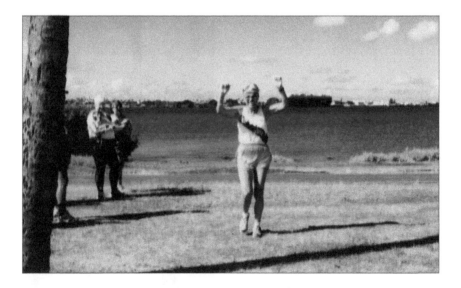

Coming in for an age-group first place at the Pearl Harbor 10K, with Pearl Harbor in the background.
August 2003.

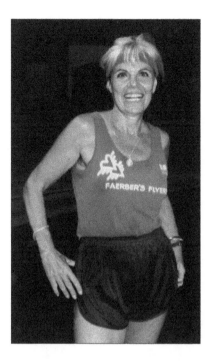

"Glowing" after a hard workout at the track.
January 1998.

With some of my hundreds of medals.

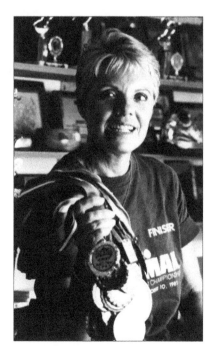

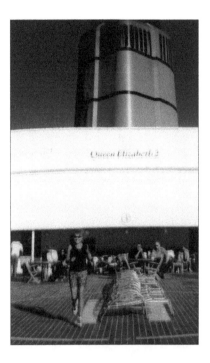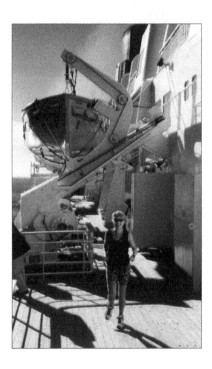

Running on board the Queen Elizabeth II *in the middle of the Atlantic. I'd taken the QE2 to London and planned to then take a flight to Istanbul to give a lecture at a conference. Then 9/11 struck and both my flight to Istanbul as well as the conference got canceled. I had to wait a whole week before I could get a flight back to the US due to the mass confusion in the immediate aftermath of 9/11.*
September 2001.

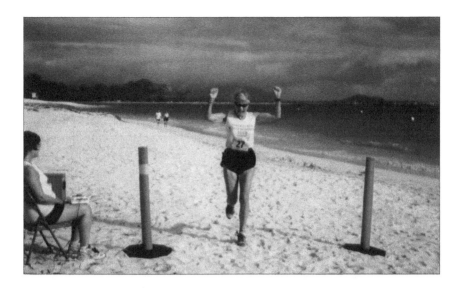

Finishing age-group first place at the Kailua Beach 5-mile race (re-enacted so as to capture the scene of one of Hawaii's most beautiful beaches).
July 2003.

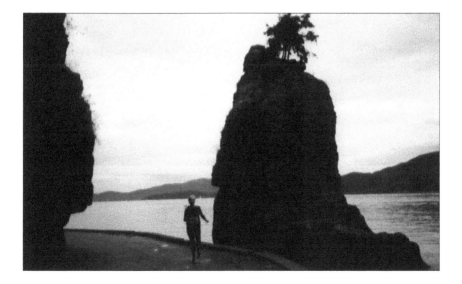

Running at Stanley Park by Siwash Rock, Vancouver, BC, Canada.
February 2003.

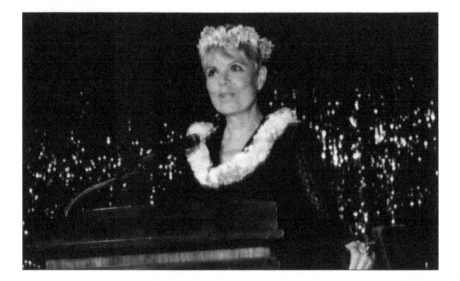

Giving the keynote speech for the opening of the Breast Care Center, Holy Cross Hospital,
South San Francisco, CA.
November 1995.

CHAPTER ELEVEN

PUTTING IT ALL TOGETHER: YOU'RE DOING A TRIATHLON

Now that you've got all three sports handled, are you ready to do a triathlon? Well, you could! These athletic events are so much fun that you'll see competitors with big smiles on their faces, especially the age-groupers. These are usually middle-of-the-packers, who are there because they enjoy the sport and want to do well primarily when competing among peers around their age.

Let's face it. If you're over forty, you really don't have much of a chance against a well-trained twenty-five-year-old. To keep the action lively for everybody, competitors are sorted into age groups, each usually with a five-year spread, such as 20–24 or 60–64. If you get an age-group first place, you'll know that you did very well when stacked up against athletes who are much more closely your equals. You will find male and female divisions as well.

Advantages of Cross-Training

The fun of competing in triathlons aside, I believe that multi-sport training is better for the body. Each sport tends to emphasize only certain muscle groups. These muscle groups can be overworked, leading to injuries and leaving other muscle groups under-exercised. Running and biking work out primarily the lower body and swimming the upper body. To be more precise, running emphasizes the hamstring muscles at the back of the thigh; cycling, the quadriceps (those bulging front thigh muscles); and swimming, the shoulders, chest, and upper arms. This is not to say that other muscle groups don't get exercised at all in each sport, because they do. It's just that they don't get exercised with nearly the same intensity. On the other hand, multi-sport training and events work out more of the whole body.

When you put the three sports—running, biking, and swimming—together, you get an excellent full-body exercise program. All three contribute to cardiovascular fitness and are excellent fat-burners. I've seen both men and women totally reshape their bodies and develop pleasing, curvaceous contours with this type of training. And you can bet that they are darned proud of their new forms. Those tight-fitting aerodynamic outfits have more than one function!

So how does the human body cope with all these different demands placed on it? Very well, thank you. Sure, there are muscle groups that tighten up while you practice one sport, but they get loosened and stretched in another. In response to increased demands on the body, blood vessels open up to support a greater supply of blood to the muscle groups being used. This happens automatically; and just as automatically, blood is redirected to the next set or sets of muscles being used.

This is why I have found that it doesn't matter in which order you do your training. Blood vessels are two-way streets, so to speak, and they will move blood to wherever the demand is. I have done back-to-back workouts in every conceivable order and have found the transition easy. As a matter of fact, although the swim is usually first in a triathlon, I love to finish my training with a swim because I can then cool down and stretch out. It's the best way to end a session!

The Importance of Transitions

In a triathlon, it is obvious that the first one to cross the finish line wins. What is not as obvious is that it is not always the fastest swimmer-cyclist-runner who crosses the finish line first. Time is required to switch from one sport to another, which is called a transition and which at times can make the difference between first place and second place. In your workouts, you will need to practice transitioning; that is, you need to rehearse switching swimming gear for cycling gear, then cycling gear for running gear.

The best way to do this is to lay out all your equipment in the transition area, with careful thought given to the order of use. As you're coming out of the water, you'll be pulling off your goggles and swim cap and thinking about what you'll do when you find your bike—which, of course, you will spot by having very strategically noted its location in relation to a landmark. Races have been lost because of "lost" bikes. Some triathlons start so early that it's still pitch dark when you're placing your bike in the rack. When you come out of the water, the scene is totally transformed, not only by the time of day but also by the sea of bikes. Know your bike's location!

Do you want to know how to tell a novice triathlete? They're the one with a bucket of water to wash the salt or sand off during the transition to the bike leg. The old hands know that it's a waste of time to shower or rinse off your feet before putting on cycling shoes. The salt does not cause chafing, and besides, you will soon be creating a salt bath with your own perspiration. Don't worry about sand or dirt on your feet from running out of the water barefoot either—it will drop right to the bottom of your socks or shoes, and you will never even know it's there. In time, you'll also find out that it's much easier to put on your bike shorts before your shoes and your cycling jersey before your helmet. And you'll know to put on your gloves and sunglasses last!

All of these considerations suggest the order in which you should place your equipment. You'll also want to have a plastic bag in which to put your swim gear. While the protection of your used equipment may not be a priority during a race, the scratching of a $50 pair of goggles can cause a lot of grief long after the race is won.

Upon returning from the cycling portion of the race, you'll need to get out of your biking shoes (unless you're a super-sport and just pull your feet out as you dismount, leaving your shoes still attached to the pedals). You can also be pulling off your gloves as you approach the transition area.

Some athletes just run in their bike shorts to save transition time. Comfort can be a very important consideration, especially if it's a particularly hot day for a long run. What have you gained if you've saved fifteen seconds in transition but your pace is five seconds per minute slower because your body is overheating? Since body temperature rises so fast during exercise, overheating is a real problem. A lot of male competitors shed their cycling jerseys for this reason.

Read All about It!

If you're a serious competitor, you're probably already subscribed to magazines on triathlons in order to keep up with what's going on in the sport. Here, you'll find a wealth of specialized information: there are whole articles just on transitions, for example. These magazines also offer an overview of new or upcoming equipment. Your neighborhood triathlon store is probably stocked with dozens of little (and some not-so-little) gadgets to help you go faster.

It's worth your time to do some serious browsing on a continual basis and to get on good terms with the store's employees, who very frequently are some of the sport's top competitors. As you pick their brains, you'll be picking up valuable tips on all aspects of training and racing. Whenever you find a new (and hopefully better) technique, you will need to try it out. It just makes good sense never to do anything different for the first time on race day. You will need to actually enact the motions of each transition. When you find the sequence that works best, then you can go through the motions mentally. Visualization is an excellent adjunct to your training. When you're out on long runs, picture in your mind how it would feel to come out of the water and have your legs re-adapt to bearing the weight of your body on a vertical instead of horizontal plane. Your mental checklist should include how you're going to replenish fluids even if you don't feel thirsty.

All this rehearsal will help you keep a cool head and not panic, irrespective of the pandemonium going on around you. I use my transition time to calm myself and run through my own mental checklist. You will usually find race volunteers in the area, ready and very willing to assist in whatever way they can. If you need help, ask calmly and specifically for what you need. I've seen competitors yelling, cursing, and throwing things at poor volunteers who could only respond with: "'It?' I don't know what 'it' is! Just tell me what you need." Pronouns do you no good if the volunteers don't know what you're referring to. In any case, they never deserve to be yelled at. They are just as excited as you are and just as anxious to get you back on the road. Use but don't abuse them!

Now, let's assume you've just gotten through your first triathlon. While everything's still fresh in your mind, write down all the lessons you've learned. If you're smart, you'll never make the same mistake twice. Since most triathletes don't do too many back-to-back races, it might be some time before you race again. To prevent feelings of panic the night before your next triathlon, make some notes on what worked and what didn't work this time. It'll save you a lot of anxiety.

Have You Hugged Your Race Director Today?

Besides the wonderful volunteers at competitions, there are race directors— self-sacrificing souls who also need to be treated right. If things have gone wrong, race directors need feedback, but preferably given in a calm, rational way. After all, if they don't have a satisfying experience, they won't be back either. Negative opinions need to be expressed with constructive comments. On the other hand, what race directors also love more than anything else is to know what went well with their race. So be a good competitor and treat everybody well!

CHAPTER TWELVE

TIME MANAGEMENT: HOW TO FIT IT ALL IN

At this point, many might wonder how to find the time to do all the things I've mentioned so far. This issue is one that I faced squarely when I started my running program back in 1968. I have always been inclined to get involved in many things at once (I always had to work while going to school, for instance), and so efficient use of my time is extremely important to me. In an effort to squeeze more into every day, I've taken several courses and read a number of books on time management, including *Getting Organized* and *How to Organize Your Life and Get Rid of Clutter*.[1,2] The main principles that I've taken from these resources and applied to my life have to do with prioritizing things to be done and getting up earlier in the morning without compromising my sleep.

At the time that I started running in 1968, I was working as a guidance counselor, going to graduate school, and raising and trying to cope with two adolescent kids. As you might guess, any extra time that I had was at a real premium. Yet, after reading Dr. Cooper's book *Aerobics*, I knew then that I had to find the time to add exercise to my life. It seemed that my new commitment to exercise would pay off in terms of not only physical benefits but also increased efficiency in my work and studies.

The only time available to me to squeeze in my running was early in the morning. By rising an hour earlier, I was able to devote that hour to getting in a good workout as well as to being alone with my thoughts. I planned my day, solved problems, experienced the joy of watching the sun rise, felt the coolness and quietness of the early morning, and returned from each run feeling euphoric, strong, lean, and healthy. I knew then that I'd found a way to handle all the stress generated from my job, graduate school, and parenthood.

No matter how busy I was, though, I always found the time to try to help other breast cancer patients by telling them what I did to cope with my horrible diagnosis. Through the auspices of the American Cancer Society's

Speaker's Bureau and its breast cancer support group Reach to Recovery, I became a volunteer speaker and would get frequent calls to visit and talk to a newly diagnosed breast cancer patient about the value of lifestyle changes, including dietary changes, in aiding recovery from cancer and lowering the risk of a recurrence. This all came to an abrupt halt, however, when one of the doctors complained to the Cancer Society that I was "interfering with the advice" given to a patient by her doctor—that she could eat anything she wanted! I'm not sure how much the situation has changed after all these years. I continue to try to educate people through my website, with an "Ask Dr. Ruth" section where people can ask me anything about diet, exercise, and lifestyle.

De-Stressing "Stress"

It was after my visit to Nepal, where I saw *real* stress (described in detail in an earlier chapter), that I came to develop my philosophy of stress. I have found that stress is a catch-all term too frequently used to explain anything inexplicable. In other words, it's a scapegoat. What I've discovered is that when our bodies are exercised strenuously every day, stress as an entity almost ceases to exist. Many of the afflictions Westerners suffer from are frequently attributed to stress: heart attacks, ulcers, high blood pressure, acne, insomnia, drug addictions, and the likes have all been thought to be caused by stress. Yet when people eat a plant-based diet and get a lot of exercise, you rarely see these health problems.

No matter how much pressure I was under—with a demanding job that required constant giving to others, with voluminous readings, term papers, grades, a master's thesis, and then a doctoral dissertation—I still had lots of energy. I know that I could have done all of this only with an exercise program that allowed me to have the space and clarity of mind to problem-solve and, at the same time, dissipated the tensions and anxieties (the "stress") that kept building up. I'd always return home from a run with a lot of gratitude for how lucky I really was, feeling ready to take on the world. So, I knew I always had to make the time to get my run in.

From my very first run, I was immediately hooked. Running became integrated into my daily routine; it was as much a part of my morning ritual as brushing my teeth. Never was there a thought of, *Should I or shouldn't I?* I was in my running shoes and out the door before I knew it. There never was an excuse like, *But I don't have the time to run.*

Running has bought me more time in that it has added energy and efficiency to my day, so I could always make time for it. "But what about biking and swimming?" you ask. Well, that took a little more planning. I already discussed biking as an exercise in a previous chapter; this is strictly about time management and environmental protection.

Since I lived about eleven miles from where I worked and had always thought commuting was a horrible waste of both time and gas, I started biking to and from work. I have to admit that at first, it seemed an almost impossible endeavor. There were too many problems: What about dealing with all the traffic? What about having to shower afterwards, to change my clothes and shoes? What about needing to put on make-up and fix my matted, sweaty hair from wearing a helmet? What about flat tires or other mechanical problems? What about what people would think? Being one of the few women at the managerial level in the male-dominated military, I had enough image problems as it was. Did I really need to be doing something that could be considered so unconventional? What about the steep hill that I lived on, that I would have to bike down at break-neck speed and bike up after a long day, when I was tired?

Handling the Gremlins

One by one, I conquered all the gremlins. I took a course in biking safety to learn how to deal with traffic. A sponge bath in the rest room took care of cleaning up after each commute. I carried a change of clothes and shoes in a backpack. I combed my hair and put on a little lipstick after arriving at work. I learned a lot about changing flat tires in a hurry and, after a series of flats, discovered vinyl tire liners, which practically eliminated the problem.

Getting home was a different story, however, since that hill took a lot longer to climb back up, but I reasoned that I was getting some hill training—something that builds power in the legs. I tackled the hill in stages. On my way home the first time, I had to walk the bike up the last part of the hill. After just a week, commuting by bike seemed so natural that I wondered how I could have made such a big deal out of it.

In committing to commuting, I also decided that it was time to give up conducting my life based on what people would think. Then I found out that their reaction, for the most part, was a mixture of incredulity and admiration. Before long, I started seeing more and more people biking to work. This is a trend that I think is accelerating as I see more bike lanes and readily available bike rentals throughout different cities. Looking at the commuters' gridlock, you can see why biking is a logical way to combine fitness and a solution to the urban transportation nightmare. I even discovered that I could get to work in less time as I didn't have to sit in heavy traffic. There's also the time that I saved by not having to schedule regular cycling workouts.

Fortunately, the problem of fitting in swim training was easier to solve. There were two swimming pools within a short walking distance from my office. I swam during my lunch hour three times a week, and in those early days, a half-mile swim seemed like a lot. As my speed increased, I increased my distance. Then, on weekends, I did a long (relative to my pool-training level at the time) ocean swim. "Long" to me used to be half a mile; now, it is five miles. It's amazing how our perceptions change.

As I started to get more serious about training and competing, I wanted to add weight training. I looked at my calendar: there were two other noontime slots, on Tuesdays and Thursdays. So, weight training got added to the schedule, and I still had evenings free, except for my two weekly distance and track workouts.

When I took a medical leave of absence after my second cancer surgery, I relished the additional time that I had and that I felt could be devoted to training. What I found out was that when I had more time, I got less efficient and did not get any more training in. I also found out that the body fulfills the demands placed on it with a self-limiting alarm. When it's forced to do too much, it rebels by sending out pain signals. These signals must be attended to; if not, injury is certain to follow.

Setting Goals: Are We Done Yet?

Another way to slice the training pie is to train by time, especially if you are traveling or in a new locale. You can set the timer so that you'll be out for one or two, even four or five hours. As long as you know that there is an end and approximately when it is, you can hang on. What happens when you don't know when or where the end is that you want to give up. In the absence of any feedback, your brain says, "This could go on forever!" and goes into a state of overwhelm. When overwhelmed, you are tempted to quit.

When I began my distance swim training, I chose to train at the half-mile course located at Ala Moana Beach Park in Honolulu. The waters there are warm and sheltered by coral reefs. For my first session, I got into the water at one end and swam for what seemed like forever. My progress was frustratingly slow. I had picked as my point of reference the high-rise building at the mid-point of the course, but once I got abreast of the building itself, the second half seemed to take even longer. When I finally reached the end of the half-mile course, I walked back.

It would take another couple of months of training before I'd gained enough strength and courage to swim both ways. The way back, of course, seemed to take forever as well. It was certainly an interesting lesson in figuring out how to handle longer distances without giving up.

The Importance of Sub-Goals

As I increased my swimming distance, I learned to take advantage of lifeguard stands. Let's say that the lifeguard stands were 200 feet apart and that there were five of them. I knew it was no problem for me to swim 200 feet—the equivalent of only eight lengths of a 25-foot pool. Upon reaching each lifeguard stand, I would then head towards the next. After a few weeks, I could swim 2,000 feet so much more easily than I had ever thought possible. This became a habit: whenever I got bored, I started counting lifeguard stands and telling myself that it was just another one or two until the end. Learning to set sub-goals like this totally changed my concept of swimming distance.

The same principle applies to indoor stationary-bicycle training, which is sometimes a necessity even in Hawaii due to heavy rain or is preferred for reasons of convenience. Rather than just get on the bike and go for as long as I can, if I set some intermediate goals, I can get through a workout of any length. Another little trick that I've learned is to do a mental count. By counting to ten on each of my fingers, I can get to a hundred repetitions of anything relatively painlessly. This is how I got through climbing up the steep hill to my house each day, standing and putting as much force as I could on my bike's pedals. You can always bear the pain for just a little bit longer when the end is in sight.

One Two, One Two: Running into Self-Hypnosis

Looking back on my training for the Ironman, I can see that what I was doing was a form of self-hypnosis, although I had no idea at the time. I'd get into a relaxed rhythm whether I was running, swimming, or cycling. Of course, all three sports are very rhythmic, following a "one two, one two" cadence.

These sports can also be very dissociative. Once you get the mechanics of running, swimming, or cycling down, your body will do it automatically and your mind will naturally wander. My mind would start to visualize scenes of triumph and excitement; I would imagine crossing the finish line of the Ironman. Without even knowing it, I was taking advantage of my "right-brain" functions.

You probably know that the human brain is said to be divided by neurological functions into the right and left sides. The left side of the brain, for most of us, is where we analyze data, exercise our time consciousness, and keep our check on reality—functions that make use of concrete, objective thinking. The right brain, on the other hand, is where we create, dream, and lose track of time. Not hampered by practical limitations, we can use the right brain to transport ourselves anywhere in space and time, from the beginning of the universe to the furthest point in the distant future. We can become anybody or anything!

It was thanks to my right brain that I started to transform my dream of conquering the Ironman into reality. Totally lost in the imaginings happening on this side of my brain, I got through longer and longer training sessions, enjoying them so much that I'd always look forward to the next. What I was doing was, in effect, giving myself positive reinforcement: I felt that my training was providing me with rewards above and beyond glowing physical health.

People with hectic schedules usually envy those who appear to have more time. They needn't. Busy people are already more efficient because they have to be organized, focused on their priorities, and on top of their schedules. I hope that this chapter dispenses with the most common excuse for not exercising. As your physical training progresses, your body becomes better able to handle greater distances. As your body becomes able to handle more, your mind leads the way by setting greater and greater goals, which make your previous ones seem easy by comparison. We must all find time to exercise. It will reward us by providing us with more quality time and greater enjoyment of the time we do have. With these lessons learned, all you have to do is go along for the ride. And what a ride it is!

You're Entitled to 120 Years!

More than 80 percent of our population dies of lifestyle-related diseases, primarily heart disease, at ages far below 120. You have it within your power to control your lifespan through lifestyle changes, primarily with respect to diet and exercise, albeit changes that may have to be drastic.

Scientific studies show that the time we invest into exercise will be rewarded back to us.[3] Training not only adds additional years to our lifespan, it also gives us a greater quality of life to the very end. The ideal is to live out our full 120 years while being active and completely self-sufficient, with all our capabilities intact.[4] We should be able to die peacefully in our sleep with little decline in our physical and mental functions. This is what happens in the famed Blue Zones.

Take a look at some of the master athletes in their eighties and nineties, even past a hundred, and you'll see what I mean. Spry of step, mentally alert, and sexually active, they are still enjoying life to its fullest. Don't know any of them? Attend some of the World Vets Championship races, the Senior Games, and the Senior Olympics, and you'll see age groups including centenarian competitors. This exercise and diet program really does work!

CHAPTER THIRTEEN

ACCIDENTS: THE CRASH I CAN'T REMEMBER

"Where am I? Where's my bike?"

As if all the medical problems related to breast cancer that I had to contend with weren't enough, I had a near-fatal bike crash that laid me up for six weeks. Since it happened only seven weeks before the Ironman, things looked pretty grim for my hope of getting to the start line.

Preparation for any race involves knowing the course. Since the Ironman was to take place on the Big Island of Hawaii, I'd gone there seven weeks before the event to practice the swim, bike ride, and run. My father, who lived there at the time, had all sorts of misgivings about my riding a bike on the roads there, believing them to be fraught with danger. It wasn't as if I thought otherwise; it was just that I was willing to take the risk, which, although I was by no means an expert cyclist, I felt was not unreasonable.

It was late August 1984; I was tooling along Queen Kaahumanu Highway, at about Mile 97 of the 112-mile course. I was just a few miles from the village of Kona. The last thing I remembered before everything went dark was passing the turn-off to the airport, excited about how good I felt and confident that I was going to be able to do the bike leg with no problems.

The next thing I remembered was being told that I was in the hospital and that it was 10:30 at night. I shifted my weight ever so slightly and felt pain shooting—quite literally—from head to toe.

I asked the nurse: "What happened? Where am I? Where's my bike?"

"We told you," she said. "Don't you remember? You're in the hospital."

A medical technologist then came in to draw my blood and started talking to me as if she knew me. I was totally confused! She laughed and said, "You've asked me at least a dozen times already, 'What happened and where's my bike?'"

"I asked *you*?" I said incredulously.

"Yes," she said, "when I drew your blood this afternoon. You were asking everybody in sight."

"But hospital personnel wouldn't know things like where my bike is," I replied.

"Well, you asked them anyway," she said. "Then, two minutes later, you asked them again, and again!"

Boy, was my mind reeling from the shock! Here I was, in a hospital, not knowing how I had gotten there, and being told that I had said things I didn't even remember saying. Slowly, I was able to piece the story together. A passing pick-up truck had grazed me, knocking me off my bike. I was found unconscious by the side of the road. A motorist who had witnessed the crash called an ambulance with his CB radio. The ambulance crew checked my vital signs and determined that I had suffered some kind of a major-impact fall and had sustained, at the minimum, a concussion, that I was not in need of an IV, and that I was going to require the services of an emergency room.

Luckily, I had had a helmet on. No, I shouldn't say "luckily." I had learned from my very first day of cycling that a helmet was an absolute necessity when riding and therefore wouldn't even go around the block without one. In my case, I had hit the ground hard enough to crack the helmet open, which could have been the fate of my head. (I was actually handed the two halves of my helmet later.) I had sustained a three-inch-long cut on the side of my head, plus the concussion. The doctors said that if I had not been wearing a helmet, there was little doubt that I would have been killed. The impact of the fall alone also sheared off the metal toe clips that had kept my feet tightly strapped to the pedals of my bike.

I tried again to shift my weight a little to get more comfortable. The sudden, stabbing pain in my right hip brought me up short. "Oh my God, the pain! What happened to my hip?" I wailed, on the verge of tears. The hospital personnel again told me that they had taken x-rays and found I'd sustained a hip fracture; they tried to assure me that I'd be fine after the six to eight weeks it would take to heal.

"But I've got an Ironman in seven weeks!" I said.

They shook their heads. "No way!"

The doctor on call when they had brought me into the ER, Dr. Frank Ferren, happened to be the medical director for the Ironman, so he was quite familiar with triathletes and the training they underwent. He'd also treated a number of bike crash victims. He shook his head too: "No way! Look, just forget it for this year. Get well and plan for next year's event."

But I had my own thoughts about what I was going to do. I'd invested too much into this venture. I felt that if breast cancer couldn't stop me, I wasn't about to let anything else keep me from doing the Ironman.

I wanted to get out of that bed and back to my training routine. I felt just like I had felt after my cancer surgeries—motivated and ready to train once more. The plotting and scheming started immediately, primarily because I didn't want all my conditioning to go down the tubes! All I could think about was getting out of there. I wanted to get back to my running, swimming, and, yes, biking.

What bothered me more than anything else was the amnesia. I could remember passing the airport road that morning, but I had been found two miles past it. I couldn't remember being hit or any of the people who had stopped to help me. I couldn't remember the ambulance ride or the emergency-room repairs—the stitching of the gash in my head, the x-rays, the blood drawing, all the bandages covering what they said were injuries from a "seven-point landing," and who knows what else. Then there was also the fact that my brain seemed to be short-circuiting, prompting me to ask the same questions repeatedly: "What happened? Where's my bike?"

The nurses seemed somewhat amused by the whole situation, but I was really upset. Why couldn't I remember? Dr. Ferren explained that what I had was both anterograde and retrograde amnesia: after a concussion, people can forget things that happened immediately prior to as well as after the impact.

As I was in the hospital for almost a week, I spent hours mentally digging through my brain cells and prodding them, *Remember, darn it, remember!* It was months later, when I was still mentally digging, that all of a sudden, I remembered some sharp, stabbing, needle-like pains. That had to be from the cut in my head being stitched up. Then I recalled a vague image of an elevator. Yes, that had to be from the ride on a gurney to my hospital room. Then I remembered three or four people trying to move me off the gurney. I obviously had not been sedated; I had screamed in pain as they lifted me up onto the bed.

The hip pain was no better a week later, when I had recovered enough to move about on crutches and fly back home to Honolulu. I had been scheduled to see an orthopedic specialist at Tripler Hospital a few days later to have a bone scan, which involved a radioactive substance being injected into my blood and, over the period of a couple of hours, settling into areas of bone injury. As it turned out, the test disclosed the hip fracture and a shattered acetabulum (the socket into which the head of the femur fits).

My first Ironman wasn't the only plan derailed by my accident. I'd previously also entered the Waikiki Roughwater Swim, which was to take place that weekend and which was important to me because it represented the first event of the Ironman. If I couldn't do the Roughwater Swim, I was in real trouble. I had never given up the idea that no matter what, I was going to be there for the start of the Ironman.

With my bone scan on the lighted screen, the orthopedic specialist shook his head and said: "No, there's definitely a fracture there. It's going to be six to eight weeks on crutches. Forget the Ironman."

Almost in desperation, I said: "What about swimming? What if I just move my upper body and not kick? Swimming should be good, shouldn't it?"

Looking at me as if I'd lost my marbles, the doctor almost pleaded: "Look, let those bones knit! If you keep moving them, you're taking a chance on permanent damage to your hip. There's a risk of necrosis! Necrosis—death of the bone!"

Now, I really *was* in trouble. How could I tell the doctor that I'd been swimming daily since getting out of the hospital? He didn't look like he'd understand if I told him how careful I was about avoiding weight-bearing movement and keeping my hip immobile, about not kicking my feet and legs at all. Thoroughly frightened and chastened, I gave up. *They're right*, I thought. *Forget it.*

That lasted until I got home. I guess the fear wore off, and I found myself scheming and figuring out how to at least start the Roughwater Swim. Because there were course marshals on surfboards all along the 2.4-mile course, I could drop out at any time if I had to.

All that was left for me to do was get somebody to take the crutches from me after I got into the water and bring them down to the end of the course, 2.4 miles away, so I could walk up the beach to the swim finish line at the end. People thought I was crazy to even think of this plan but finally relented when they saw that I was determined to swim in the race, with or without their help. (A photo of the finish is included in the photo section.)

And so it was in 1984 that I learned that swimming for a triathlete is a primarily upper-body sport. I found that my time was not that much slower, that my dragging legs still acted as a rudder, and that I could do things that I "shouldn't" if I wanted to badly enough.

Now, this is not to say that the doctors were wrong. The safest course, surely, is to always rest and recover after an injury. It's just that you're taking a chance if you persist in training, even if at a lower level, in the face of an injury. I was really lucky, and in fact, I healed much faster than the medical estimates indicated I would. I know that it wasn't as much luck as it was my healthy diet that contributed to the fast recovery. I was off the crutches in four weeks instead of the predicted six to eight weeks. Having undergone eight surgeries now and a whole lot of injuries, I can confidently say that the fit vegan athlete heals much faster than does the average, sedentary person.

Healing Fast

The rest of my recovery proceeded at an accelerated pace. After the Roughwater Swim, I started toying with the idea of getting on my stationary bicycle. I argued with myself for another week and then thought: *What the heck! If it hurts, I'll just stop.* Sure enough, after just a couple of minutes on the stationary bike, it did start to hurt. I did not persist. I wasn't really disappointed or depressed either, though. I resolved to just keep checking every day until it was all good, and I knew that I'd know exactly when that was. The next morning, thinking that I'd had another twenty-four hours of healing time, I felt bold. Time to try again!

To my surprise, I could go four minutes before pain set in. On the third day, my time doubled again. I got very excited as I computed my recovery rate. I already knew that I had the swim of the Ironman handled; now, it looked as though I might possibly be okay to complete the bike leg too. Sure enough, each day, I saw tremendous improvement. Coincidentally, besides the Waikiki Roughwater Swim, I had long ago also entered in the *Honolulu Advertiser*'s Century Ride—which was now going to be just five weeks from the accident. Here was my chance to see if could do a 100-miler on the bike. To my greatest surprise and delight, I made it through the entire 100 miles without too much pain. I now knew without a shadow of doubt that I was going to go for at least the first two parts of the Ironman.

On my next medical check-up, five weeks after the crash, I told the doctor that I thought I was healing way ahead of schedule. After poking and prodding, seeing that I was not yelling out in pain, he appeared satisfied.

He backed away, putting his hands on his hips. "Let's see if you can walk," he said. It had been a whole week in the hospital and four weeks on crutches. I almost panicked.

"*Walk?*" I asked, wide-eyed.

I suddenly got cold feet. I had grown attached to those crutches and was not sure I was ready for the real showdown. What if I *couldn't* walk? The Ironman was now only two weeks away. I slowly, carefully put a little weight on my right foot, the side of the hip fracture. It seemed okay so far. I put a little more weight on that foot: still okay. The doctor held out a steadying hand, and I put all my weight on that foot.

"Oh my God!" I whooped. I was standing and nothing hurt! Another slow series of weight transfers, this time to the left foot. And still no pain! Another step, and another. I let the joy sink in, "I'm okay . . . I'm okay!"

"All right now, just take it easy," the doctor said. "You've still got quite a bit of healing to do. Don't get over-exuberant and do too much."

The next day, I was able to walk (even run very slowly) for almost two minutes. Unbeknownst to me, I was about to discover that getting back to running was just like getting back to biking. However, the Ironman was now only thirteen days away; I was going to have to run a full marathon then. I couldn't keep doubling my time, so I stopped a week before the race with a single twelve-mile run. At that point, I didn't care what would happen; however it worked out, I told myself, I would be there at the start line and would go as far as I could.

Amazingly, I had a wonderful first Ironman. Because of all that had occurred in the previous seven weeks, survival was all that was on my mind. There was not even the slightest wish to *race*. That, as it turned out, was the best thing that could happen. I was forced to pace myself; as a result, I finished in 14 hours and 49 minutes, well before the final cut-off time of 17 hours, feeling totally amazed that I was even able to accomplish this feat. As I crossed the finish line and saw Dr. Ferren, he said, "If I hadn't seen this myself, I wouldn't have believed it!"

The official results weren't available until the next morning. When I saw that I was just one minute from placing in the 45–49 age group, I was so excited that I immediately started plotting a new training schedule. *Just think what I could have done if I had been able to train for the last seven weeks,* I mused. *Just wait until next year, when I'll be fifty!* That would put me in a new age group, 50–54. It would help to be the youngest in an age group instead of the oldest, which I had been.

Now, if I could only remember that ambulance ride!

Truck–Bike Accident Number Two

Back in 1998, while training to enter the Australian Ironman, I was on a 25-mile bike ride out to Hawaii Kai. At one point, I had the choice of taking the busy main highway or the side roads. I took the latter, figuring it would be a lot safer. Boy, did I get that wrong!

As I approached an intersection, a truck loaded with kitchen cabinets did the same on the opposite side. The driver was looking for a street to turn onto that was on the left, but since street signs were on the right, that was where he was looking. When he saw that it was his street, he made an impulsive, immediate left turn. The problem is that I was in the middle of the intersection, and he T-boned me. I went flying off the bike, landing flat on my back a few feet away. Never losing consciousness, I knew that the accident was serious from the extreme pain in both my left leg and right hip. I looked down at my left leg and didn't like what I saw. Though there was no blood, there was an ominous bump that looked like bone.

I heard the driver exclaim, "I never even saw her!" then another voice, "I just called 911." A nice gentleman put a pillow under my head and shielded me from the bright noonday sun. Almost immediately, it seemed, I heard sirens. An ambulance pulled up; two attendants jumped out, started asking me questions, and proceeded to load me up onto a stretcher and into the ambulance. One of them said: "You were lucky. We were just a block away." I told them I was a Kaiser patient, thinking that this way, they'd have my medical records. "No way!" was the response. "You're going to the major trauma center at Queen's Hospital."

When I got to the emergency room, they took x-rays and came back with the devastating news. My left tibia was shattered and the right side of my pelvis was fractured in three places. The only good news about the pelvic fractures was that they were non-displaced, meaning no surgery. This warranted a diagnosis of multifocal fractures—fractures on both sides of my body—which meant absolutely *no* weight bearing until they healed. I was taken upstairs to the orthopedics ward and put in a special orthopedic bed with two monkey bars (hanging rings) above me so I could pull myself up when I needed to use a bed pan.

Later that evening, I was paid a visit by the orthopedic doctor on call, Dr. Jay Marumoto. He said that he'd ordered some pain medication for me since they had determined it was safe to do so. He told me that given my x-rays, I had two options. The first was to allow him to put a tibial rod in my left leg so that I could at least, with crutches, start some weight bearing on that leg. He described what would be a very scary surgery. There would be blood and bone marrow splattering all over the operating room, as he would have to drill through the center of my tibia (shin bone) to allow him to insert a twelve-inch-long titanium rod reaching from my ankle to my knee. When he saw my (undoubtedly horrified) expression upon hearing this description, Dr. Marumoto said that my only other alternative was to stay in bed for six to eight weeks. He concluded, "Think about it and let me know what you want to do." And with that, he left me to deal with this agonizing choice.

I went over and over my options, going back and forth between them, unable to decide what to do. I desperately searched for a third option but none came up. When a nurse came in with the pain medication that Dr. Marumoto had ordered, I asked for her opinion. She agreed that it was a tough decision, that either way, I had a long road of healing ahead of me. I didn't get much sleep that night, nor did morning bring any answers.

When Dr. Marumoto came in the next morning on his medical rounds, I still hadn't made up my mind. I called up two friends who were medical doctors, and their consensus was that neither option had a clear advantage over the other, both confirming that I had a tough decision to make. Feeling even more uncertain, I kept oscillating between my two only choices, unable to stick with one or the other for more than a minute or two. More importantly, I knew I had to decide soon because I suspected I was already starting to lose the fitness I had worked so hard to gain.

Later that afternoon, as I looked up at the monkey bars above my bed, a thought occurred to me: *Aha! I'm going to do whatever upper-body exercise is possible.* I started to do a pull-up. Right at that moment, one of the nurses walked in. "What in the world are you doing?" she gasped. I told her that I was trying to at least keep some upper-body fitness.

Two whole days went by and still no decision. On the evening of the third day, a nurse came in with some forms, laid them down on my tray table, and started to walk out. "Wait, what are these?" I asked. She told me that they were permits for Dr. Marumoto to perform the surgery in the morning. She left. I realized that they had made the decision for me. Now, the only way I could object was to not sign the forms. I swallowed really hard and put down my signature.

I was on so many drugs that my memories of those days are faint. I do remember being told the surgery had gone well. I also remember being given a morphine pump that allowed me to decide how much pain I could handle during recovery—a medical godsend thanks to which I could then handle the twice-daily physical therapy, starting on a very long journey to rehabilitation.

When I was discharged from the hospital nearly three weeks later, I had a prescription for physical therapy three times a week—on Monday, Wednesday, and Friday. I found it so helpful that I asked if I could increase the number of weekly sessions to five, adding Tuesday and Thursday. Insurance would not cover the extra sessions, so I paid for them myself. The physical therapy was *that* valuable.

I recalled the stages of recovery that I'd gone through the first time I'd been hit by a truck. Once again, I got back into the water for water running and swimming, back onto the stationary bike, and gradually back onto my feet to run. I decided to do all my biking on the stationary bike, having gotten a taste of how risky it was to do a lot of training on roads. Let me serve as an example of why you should always wear a helmet: no matter how skillful you are on the bike, your skills can't save you from careless drivers.

Later on, I turned to spin classes as they provided a lot of high-intensity training. In fact, that was all the bike training I did before competing in both the State and National Senior Olympics, winning a total of eight gold medals.

Needless to say, I had to take a pass on the Australian Ironman.

CHAPTER FOURTEEN

ARTHRITIS: DIET DOES MAKE A DIFFERENCE

Despite my athletic accomplishments, one of my central beliefs is that this body of mine is fairly average and that it responds to good and bad things done to it just as yours would. While I recognize that there are individual differences, they are outnumbered by the similarities that we as humans all share, as I've suggested elsewhere. If we took just our skeletons and hung them up side by side, they'd all look nearly identical and you'd have trouble telling them apart. If we weren't so similar, we would not be able to have the same blood test done and know if the results fall within the "normal" ranges. Radiologists would be surprised each time they look at an x-ray because our x-rays would look wildly different. Of course, this is not the case; we are all rather predictable.

You probably are aware that arthritis is a fairly common malady: maybe you've been asked to donate to the Arthritis Foundation in order to search for a cure, or you've read articles in newspapers and magazines about the different types of arthritis. Most of us know people who are afflicted with this painful joint disease, which often leads to total joint replacements. We are told that it's not just a common but an expected part of aging (at least in the case of degenerative osteoarthritic or so-called wear-and-tear arthritis), that there's no cure, and that diet does not affect arthritis one way or the other.

When I hit forty-two years of age in 1977, I went to see a doctor because of the gradual onset of stiffness and pain in my back. Waking up in the morning, I could hardly bend over. I had to use both hands, hanging onto the walls, to lower myself down to the toilet. And it took me about ten minutes of gradual movement to loosen my back enough to put my shoes on.

X-rays were taken and a hands-on examination was performed. The doctor's verdict was osteoarthritis. I was told that it was nothing serious and just part of growing older. My running, according to this doctor, was probably aggravating it, and I should just resign myself to the inevitable.

He added that there was nothing I could do to alleviate it, though there was a new drug that had just come onto the market, a non-steroidal anti-inflammatory called naproxen, that should ease the discomfort. It was not a cure, however, so I'd probably have to take it for the rest of my life. Of course, there was no mention of the possible side effects of long-term use such as cartilage damage, erosion of the stomach lining, hemorrhage, constipation, and more.

The pills seemed great! I woke up each morning totally flexible and able to move without pain; I thought wonderful things about the "miracles" of modern medicine. During the ensuing years, I'd periodically be asked by doctors if I was on any medication, and I'd say that I wasn't because I didn't even think of naproxen as medication or a drug. Taking naproxen had become such a "normal" part of my life that it was just like taking a vitamin pill.

Then came one of the side effects, the erosion of my stomach lining. This was causing a significant amount of gastrointestinal (GI) bleeding that ultimately led me to the emergency room (described in detail in the chapter on anemia). When the doctors asked me the standard question, I again gave my usual answer, "No medications."

After receiving a diagnosis of iron-deficiency anemia, I called my "diet doctor," Dr. McDougall; I told him where I was calling from and that the doctors were blaming my meatless diet for my not getting enough iron. After all, they "knew" that red meat provides heme iron, the "best" source of iron. (We now know that this is not true at all.)[1]

Dr. McDougall assured me that if I was suffering from iron-deficiency anemia, I could be sure I was losing blood from somewhere. I told him that I did have black stools periodically, after long, hard races. His guess was GI bleeding. He then asked me, "You aren't taking any medication, are you?" I was starting to give my automatic reply when I suddenly realized my error.

"Whoa, yes!" I said. "I completely forgot about naproxen. I've been taking that for years now."

"Why in the world are you taking *that* drug?" he asked.

"For my arthritis!" I replied.

"You don't have arthritis. It went away when you changed your diet. It's probably the naproxen that's causing your GI bleeding!"

Taking heed of Dr. McDougall's words, I immediately stopped the pills, anticipating the return of the back pain and stiffness of my pre-naproxen days. To my surprise and delight, there was not even a hint of discomfort. Dr. McDougall, on the other hand, was not surprised in the least, proclaiming, "Despite what the Arthritis Foundation claims, diet *does* make a difference!"

Apparently, when I changed my diet due to my cancer, I also inadvertently did the best thing possible for my osteoarthritis. A recent study has shown NSAIDS—common non-steroidal, anti-inflammatory drugs like the one prescribed to me—work by inhibiting hormones called prostaglandins. This process can actually cause the opposite of the desired effect: it can destroy joint tissue more so than the osteoarthritis itself.[2]

Another interesting fact is that the incidence of osteoarthritis follows the same pattern in relation to diet as do incidences of all the common cancers and degenerative diseases. Inflammatory arthritis is most common in countries whose populations eat the Western diet and rarest in countries whose populations eat a low-fat, plant-based diet. Again, this difference is not attributable to heredity, because when people migrate to the US and adopt the SAD or Western diet, they soon get osteoarthritis at the same rate as does the rest of the US population. This has been shown to be true even with rheumatoid arthritis.[3]

Why is this? The theory has to do with the reaction of animal proteins in the human body. Once animal proteins leak into the bloodstream, the body's immune system forms antibodies against them as it would against any foreign protein. In people prone to arthritis, these immune complexes are filtered out of the bloodstream and end up in the joints. Here, they act like tiny slivers of wood, causing pain as well as swelling and inflammation of the joints. In the years after I quit naproxen, I had no arthritic symptoms in my back or anywhere else—and this after a medical doctor's prediction that I would be on arthritis medication for the rest of my life.

I also believe that the strenuous exercise program I'm on helps. When the muscles supporting one or both sides of a joint are weak, they create too much stress on the joint surfaces. Conversely, when those muscles are very strong, they support the joint structures and protect them from unnatural wear and tear. In *Aerobics*, Dr. Cooper talks about the importance of having strong abdominal and back muscles to support the spinal column.[4]

Running will build these muscles; that's why I believe it was responsible for the elimination of the terrible backaches I had had in the years before I started a running program.

Of course, there are other exercises that strengthen the back and other joints. If you are suffering from backaches, consult a physical therapist for recommendations on the most effective exercises that will help you build a strong core. All you need to do is find a routine you enjoy and eliminate all animal products from your diet, and your joint aches and pains may be a thing of the past.

Chapter Fifteen

Osteoporosis: A Hidden Handicap

I'm sitting at my not-too-user-friendly computer. Sipping my coffee substitute—a spoonful of organic blackstrap molasses dissolved in a cup of hot water—I am providing my body with the material needed to maintain and build strong bones. This delicious brew gives me a healthful bonus of 131 mg of calcium, 395 mg of potassium, 42 mg of magnesium, and 3 mg of iron. Moreover, I get to avoid the negative effects of heavy coffee drinking, defined as consuming more than five or six cups a day. A 1990 study of 101,774 subjects, even after allowing for other important risk factors such as heavy smoking and high blood pressure, showed that heavy coffee drinking increases the risk of dying of heart disease.[1] Coffee contains a central nervous system stimulant that can act as an immune depressant afterwards, and heavy coffee drinkers have been discovered to have higher levels of cholesterol than do those who drink more moderate amounts.[2] And most relevant to this chapter is the fact that because of its acidity, coffee, when drunk in excess, can rob calcium from the bones. (By comparison, soft drinks also contribute to bone loss when they contain phosphoric acid.)[3]

Milk Does Not Do a Body Good!

You may recall the "milk mustache" ads featuring prominent athletes and the motto "Milk does a body good"—part of a campaign to boost the sales of dairy, which were sagging despite many dietary recommendations perpetuating the misconception that just because milk has calcium in it, this calcium goes to the bones. When that didn't work, new ads for yogurt came out. Indeed, an Irish study of almost 2,000 men and women showed that one serving of yogurt daily lowers the risk of osteoporosis or osteopenia (low bone density, the precursor to osteoporosis and bone fractures). But those who just drank milk and ate cheese saw no bone-strengthening effect, so it turns out that it's not the calcium but the culture of probiotics in yogurt that is beneficial. And there are many other, more healthful sources of probiotics such as kimchi and sauerkraut.

One cannot escape the flood of advertisements extolling the virtues of calcium-rich dairy. Yes, of course, calcium is important. But why is it that the strongest bones in the world are found in people who supposedly have the "worst" diets, with no dairy products? Why is it that the people who eat the most dairy products have the highest incidence of osteoporosis?[4] And how did it get ordained that cattle were to be the suppliers of our calcium? Why do we not consume horse's milk, dog's milk, or even whale's milk? Even rat's milk has much more calcium per ounce than does cow's milk. When you stop to think about the purpose of an animal's milk production, obviously, it is to supply her own newborn with uniquely formulated sustenance until the latter can procure his own food. Each species' milk has a different nutritional profile depending on how fast that species' young grow. Human beings are the only species to drink the breast secretions of another species. Isn't it about time we got *weaned*?

We frequently hear that someone "fell and broke their hip"; in fact, their hip broke, which caused them to fall. Or we may hear someone claim that they just sneezed and broke a rib. There's something drastically wrong here, since it seems logical to assume that bones are supposed to last a lifetime, just as they do in the Blue Zones.

Studies show, for example, that vegetarian women have stronger bones than do meat-eating women,[5] that tennis players have much denser bones (by 35 percent) in their tennis-playing arms versus their non-playing arms and both tennis players and swimmers have greater bone density compared to non-exercising controls.[6] These results contribute to the wealth of convincing evidence that both diet and exercise are important in growing and maintaining strong, dense bones.

It is frequently said that genetics plays a role in the development of osteoporosis. This is true to the extent that we can be more or less predisposed to the effects of too much protein in our diets or too little exercise. On the other hand, it has been abundantly shown that when people with strong, dense bones from other parts of the world migrate to the US and consume the typical Western diet, they start showing signs of osteopenia or osteoporosis.

There's also the myth that pregnant and lactating women need to drink cow's milk to be able to provide enough breast milk so that their babies grow to be strong and healthy. Since a majority of the world's population has never been accustomed to consuming dairy products, it seems ridiculous that the medical profession as a whole and the USDA still actively promote dairy consumption. (Look to the lobbyists here.) In addition, there is a great deal of evidence that cow's milk causes a host of other problems, such as middle-ear infections, constipation, type 1 diabetes, food sensitivities, asthma, acne, allergies, and precocious sexual development in children from excess dietary protein.

What's the role of something like an Ironman triathlon in fighting osteoporosis? Well, can you think of a better way to build strong bones than to exercise in not one, not two, but three sports? Swimming and cycling, though low-impact (or no-impact) sports, still require your muscles to pull on your tendons, which in turn pull on your bones. These forces are enough to keep your bones strong and counteract the processes that tend to tear them down during their constant remodeling.

As students of anatomy and physiology know, there is a basic principle called Wolff's Law that says, in effect, that bones grow to be as strong as the body needs them to be. Bones are active and alive; they are, in fact, among the most active tissues in the body. Cells called osteoclasts tear down old bone to make room for new bone, built by cells called osteoblasts. These processes cause a continuous exchange of bony material in response to the demands placed on the body's bones. When people are diagnosed with osteopenia or osteoporosis, usually after having their bone density measured via a DEXA (dual-energy x-ray absorptiometry) scan, they may be put on bone-building drugs, which work by paralyzing osteoclasts, making bones *appear* denser. Actually, it's the continuous exchange between osteoblasts and osteoclasts that keeps bones strong, and these drugs only make bones more brittle and increase the risk of certain types of fracture, namely that of the femur and jaw bone. The FDA has required a labeling change to reflect this greater risk.[7]

Even more effective in building bone mass is movement that involves running and jumping, although its benefits seem to be limited primarily to the lower body and spine. Since the most serious and disabling fractures resulting from osteoporosis are in the hips and spine, running is a great anti-osteoporosis exercise, ideally accompanied by a diet conducive to building strong bones and preventing the disease from ever occurring.

In addition, bone modeling and remodeling can be positively influenced by hormones, and not to mention vitamin D. But since most of us can do little about our hormonal status and don't care to get more sun exposure than is necessary or convenient, diet and exercise are our two most viable options to ensure our bone health. You can occasionally consult an endocrinologist to test your levels of estrogen and progesterone, hormones that affect your bones.

One of the many marvels of the human body has to do with the intestinal tract, specifically the villi, which is able to take exactly what it needs from ingested food. For example, it is known that when the body is anemic, more iron is absorbed from the food passing through the intestinal tract, as measured by the total iron-binding capacity (TIBC) test. It makes perfect sense—when we need more iron, we absorb more. There is no such neat little test to tell us how much calcium we are absorbing, but it is reasonable to assume that when we need more calcium, our bodies absorb more calcium as well. This explains why older women in Africa, who get only 200–400 mg of calcium a day, have strong, dense bones even after twenty-something years of multiple pregnancies and long lactation periods.

Calcium-Pill Deficiency?

For all of the reasons noted above, we can see that osteoporosis is not due to a calcium-pill deficiency and that we don't need calcium pills to build strong bones. Additionally, studies have shown that for people who already have osteoporosis, calcium pills do them no good. Indeed, even gorging on high-calcium foods does not help people lose less bone compared to those with a lower calcium intake.[8] Likewise, post-menopausal women are frequently prescribed estrogen to try to slow down bone loss, but not all women can or want to take estrogen. Notably, for women with estrogen-receptor-positive breast cancer, taking estrogen would be like adding gasoline to the cancerous fire. On the other hand, natural progesterone, not the synthetic version in drugs such as progestin, can help reverse osteoporosis without the risk of breast or uterine cancer and is even thought to be beneficial for breast cancer patients.

As a precaution, I did periodically get DEXA scans taken to measure my bone density; apparently, my regime was working until a complicating factor developed, which will be discussed in a later chapter. During my fifties and sixties, I was at the top of the charts, with my readings exceeding that of the average thirty-year-old woman at peak bone density. The average thirty-year-old woman at peak bone density has a bone-density measurement of 411 mg/cm^2, while mine went from 447 mg/cm^2 at age fifty to 466 mg/cm^2 at age sixty!

A Hidden Handicap

I called osteoporosis a hidden handicap because so many women from age thirty-five onwards are going around with bones that are losing significant density. They have no idea that they are heading for fractures, height shrinkage, rib cages that rest on their hipbones, and dowager's humps.

With all the fuss about women not getting enough calcium, it may come as a surprise to some that men are also vulnerable to osteoporosis. Although they do not suffer the abrupt drop in sex hormone levels that women do, their hormones do lessen with time, which, combined with the negative influences of not enough exercise and a high-protein diet, puts them into a negative calcium balance. Luckily for men, they start out with denser bones, which is why they are much older before they start experiencing hip fractures, loss of height, and dowager's humps.

* * *

For three years, I was racing every weekend, sometimes taking on two or three races in a weekend. In my eagerness to improve, coupled with my love of running, I once even took part in a 25K race (and set a new state record) the week after completing an Ironman. During this time, I had a number of stress fractures—nine, to be exact. Skeptics would say that my system was not working, that I had osteoporosis and needed to drink cow's milk. I have to admit that I questioned my regime at first.

After a little research, however, I reached the conclusion that I was over-training and racing without allowing myself enough recovery time. No wonder I was having stress fractures, I was told. As I would find out, a general rule of thumb is to take one easy training day for every mile of strenuous racing. I'd never been able to come even close to that. After the fractures, my energy levels continued to be high and everything else recovered quickly. Ever since, I've backed off on strenuous runs soon after hard races. I've sustained no more stress fractures.

An interesting fact about fractures is that once a fracture is healed, a callus is formed at the site of the break that keeps it stronger than the surrounding bone for years. I never had to worry about recurring stress fractures, only about how many bones weren't able to take the load I was putting on them. It's now been many years since my last stress fracture, and my bone density not only remained stellar but even increased significantly from age fifty to sixty, according to the tests. In order to ensure that I get adequate amounts of calcium and all the other minerals that go into making bone, I continue to eat mineral-rich foods daily, including a lot of leafy greens—kale, Swiss chard, dandelion greens, cilantro, and mixed baby greens—even in my breakfast!

High Protein Can Mean Weak Bones!

America has a long-standing love affair with protein. I would venture to guess that most people still assume meat is the only source of protein, just as dairy and whey protein are the "only" source of calcium. Sadly, the US government's heavy subsidization of both meat and dairy has far-reaching consequences, affecting even school lunch programs. For years now, foods have been marketed as being high in protein because the label sells. There are high-protein supplements in the form of pills, powders, and drinks; high-protein cosmetics; high-protein anything and everything!

So what happens when you eat too much protein? Your body cannot store the excess amount. If it could, taking all those protein supplements would have you looking like Arnold Schwarzenegger by now. Although the returns are not all in yet, it appears that excess protein (characteristic of the SAD diet) is a major culprit in draining calcium from the bones. A high-protein diet is highly acidic (think of all the amino acids), and those acids must be neutralized by calcium (a base, which is alkaline by nature) to keep the blood alkaline at around the ideal pH of 7.4. The body draws calcium from the blood; then, to replenish the supply in the blood, the body draws it from the bones. Thus, the high-protein SAD diet, coupled with a sedentary lifestyle, predisposes Americans to a condition of weakened, fragile bones, just as muscles atrophy from lack of use.

An occasional excess of protein is not critical, but when people eat high-protein meals three times a day, twenty-one times a week, the effect is cumulative. Consider the Eskimos, who get plenty of protein and up to 2,500 mg of calcium a day, who also suffer from an extremely high incidence of osteoporosis at an early age.[9] By comparison, women in their twenties in the West have been diagnosed with osteoporosis. A single fast-food burger, high in protein and sodium and low in calcium, can cause the *loss* of 22 mg of calcium.[10] On the contrary, numerous studies provide evidence that plant protein does not cause calcium excretion.

Men are not immune from osteoporosis. Although it usually starts later in life for men, osteoporosis can still be a crippling disease. It can cause falls, leaving a person with a fractured pelvis or femur and totally bedridden. Once bedridden, they cannot work their bones through weight-bearing activity, which in turn rapidly accelerates bone loss. The result is a downward spiral that is often nearly impossible to reverse.

These losses from lack of weight bearing are not insignificant. Astronauts in outer space suffer measurable bone loss due to the absence of gravity pulling on their bones. Knowing this, they make an effort to get enough exercise while on a mission. Shannon Lucid, for example, exercised for an average of 2.7 hours a day while in space. She couldn't use weights because "they'd float like a feather." There was a treadmill, but with no gravity, she had to keep her feet on the treadmill by tying herself to it with a harness and bungee cords.[11]

Is Bone Broth Good for Your Bones?

Bone broth sounds like it ought to be good for building bone, right? Bone broth is made by boiling the bones of farmed animals down to get the constituents of bone, minerals from the marrow, collagen, and all the essential amino acids. The assumption is that drinking this concoction will automatically help one build more bone. Well, would you eat hair to keep from going bald? I think not! Among the facts not mentioned by bone-broth sellers is that broth made from chicken bones was found to have markedly high lead concentrations, up to ten times the control value for tap water. Studies have shown that farmed animals will sequester lead, which can be released into bone broth during its preparation.[12] In addition, every one of the minerals and amino acids in the bones of animals comes from the same original source: plants. Best to go straight to the source and avoid all the heavy-metal contamination.

Want to Shake Things Up?

One exciting new advancement that can aid in building bone density for those with osteoporosis or osteopenia is whole-body vibration. Small vibrations generated by machines are used to create instability in the body, to which muscles respond by subconsciously contracting to stabilize it. Rapid cycles of contraction and release strengthen and tone the muscles. Research has shown that when you stand on a plate that vibrates at 30 hertz/second or more, the tiny tri-planar movements stimulate your osteoblasts to build more bone.[13] A course of whole-body vibration can increase bone density as much as osteoporosis drugs can, without all the side effects. As an added bonus, a study claims that the massage function of whole-body vibration increases skin blood flow, improving skin tone and decreasing the appearance of cellulite.[14] Yet another study shows an increase in human growth hormone, which can have far-reaching positive effects on proprioception, balance, and fall prevention.[15] An internet search will yield much more recent research on this topic.

Take heed: the health of your bones is another good reason to get a lot of exercise and eat a whole-food, plant-based diet!

CHAPTER SIXTEEN

ANEMIA AND THE VEGAN DIET

One of the more interesting aspects of my journey to becoming an Ironman has been the opportunity to learn a lot about my body and the human body in general. As I upped my training levels in running by taking part in ultra-marathons, I started to notice increasing fatigue. "Isn't this normal?" you may ask. No, not in this case. Besides the fatigue, I noticed that after a long, hard run or race, I would experience light-headedness. Right after crossing the finish line of my first 50K race, I nearly passed out. Knowing enough to get my head down to keep from fainting, I darted towards the curb of the street and quickly put my head between my knees.

My thought at this time was, *Wow, I guess I'm really pushing my limits!* I felt that my light-headedness was to be expected and no real cause for alarm. When I went to stand up again a few minutes later, however, I nearly passed out again. I started to get a little concerned: it was close to midnight and I had to drive myself home.

The race director brought me some food and water that I quickly downed, thinking that my blood sugar must've gotten too low. After a few more minutes, I felt much better. I climbed into my car; I made it home and went straight to bed. The next morning, when I woke up, I still felt light-headed and close to fainting. Furthermore, I discovered that I had melena—black, tarry stools—the hallmark of gastrointestinal (GI) bleeding. Upon calling the emergency room of the now-familiar Tripler Hospital and describing my symptoms, I was told, "Get yourself into competent medical care—*now!*" I realized it must be pretty serious. These symptoms could be life-threatening, the hospital staff emphasized. They immediately assumed that it was my distance running that was causing my internal bleeding.

When I arrived at the ER, one of the first things they did was try to put a nasogastric tube into my stomach. By far the most unpleasant of all the medical procedures I've ever had done, this involves sticking a tube lubricated with K-Y jelly into a nostril, trying to miss the trachea while aiming for the esophagus. You probably know that the trachea leads to the lungs and, if blocked, makes it impossible to breathe—a feeling that causes extreme panic. Well, wouldn't you know it? It was my trachea that they hit. With the tube totally blocking the entrance to my trachea, I started gagging and struggled to breathe. I panicked and started to swing my arms wildly. They quickly pulled the tube out and apologized profusely.

They said that they needed to try again, but I was too badly shaken. I refused. No amount of pleading would change my mind, so they brought in some reinforcements. The chief of the ER said that I could be bleeding to death and that this was the only way to see what was going on.

I told him that I was sure I wasn't bleeding to death, and besides, I had to leave to get to my track workout. The doctor looked aghast! "You're not going anywhere," he said. "You don't seem to realize the seriousness of the situation. We are going to have to hospitalize you. We have to find the source of the bleeding. Now, I know what you just went through was extremely unpleasant, but we've got more experienced people who will not miss this time."

I was in turmoil. I sat there for a long time trying to reason things out. If the doctor was right, I would need to agree to let them try the procedure again. I thought about the near-fainting spells and the melena. Then the panicky feelings recreated themselves. The doctor watched as I weighed the pros and cons.

Taking my hand, he said gently: "I will do my best to minimize the discomfort. We've *got* to find the source of the bleeding."

I resigned myself to what seemed like the inevitable. This time, the doctor hit my esophagus and fed the tube into my stomach. Attaching a syringe to the other end of the tube, he started aspirating the contents of my stomach. In spite of the discomfort of having a tube through my nose and down my throat into my stomach, I watched, wide-eyed and intrigued by what was going on. What was coming out of my stomach looked like coffee grounds.

"Uh-oh," he declared. "That's bad news. You're bleeding from the stomach. There'll be no track workout today. We're keeping you right here!"

Instead of my life flashing before my eyes as the saying goes, a vision of my next race, which happened to be the Boston Marathon, went flying by. When the results of my blood tests came back from the lab, I was told that I was extremely anemic. My hemoglobin was 6.8, hematocrit 24, serum ferritin iron stores a very low 6, and total iron-binding capacity (TIBC) 399. According to the doctor, what all of this meant was that I should be flat on my back, getting a blood transfusion. (See Appendix One for an explanation of the laboratory tests.) The situation was serious. I was supposed to board a plane to Boston in two days to run the Boston Marathon. All runners know that Boston is the holy grail. I had worked too hard to qualify and was not giving it up.

I begged and I pleaded. "Look, I just finished a 50K run. If I were in as bad shape as you say, I wouldn't have been able to do that."

The doctor shook his head. "I don't know how you did it, but you are risking damage to your heart muscle by insisting on running another marathon. When you're this anemic, your blood can't carry enough oxygen to support the demands of a marathon on your heart. You're crazy to even consider it."

As you may recall from an earlier chapter, after being diagnosed with anemia, I asked if I could call Dr. McDougall, who assured me that it was likely the naproxen that was the cause of my GI bleeding. I got off the phone resolved to ditch the naproxen and feeling more relaxed. After all, I was exercising for fitness and to beat cancer; it didn't make sense to create damage to my heart while trying to get stronger. I skipped the track workout and spent the night in the Tripler Hotel.

The next day, I was "scoped," meaning that I had an endoscope passed into my stomach and upper intestine to let the doctors see what condition my GI tract was in. To my surprise and delight, everything appeared normal. As I questioned how this could be, I was told that the lining of the GI tract heals very rapidly, sometimes in fewer than twenty-four hours. They even showed me Polaroid photos of my insides. Yep, completely healed.

The doctors were very surprised at such a quick recovery and released me from the hospital with a load of iron pills. That's when a devious thought crept into my head: *Do it! Do Boston!*

I dismissed the thought.

Yes, you can, it said again.

Hmmmm, I can always stop anytime during the race, I mused. *Yes! That's it! I'm going to Boston, and I will at least start the race.* Armed with my iron pills, I arrived at the start of one of the most prestigious races in the world, thrilled to even be there. I ran the race slowly and carefully, monitoring my body signals all the way. The only real symptom I noticed was that I was really cold. I didn't think too much about it as the temperature was in the low thirties and all I was wearing was my running singlet and shorts. I put on the gloves that I'd brought and wrapped myself in a plastic garbage bag that a kind soul had given me.

My racing singlet read HAWAII across the front, which of course was not visible through the bag. I figured that after a few miles, when I'd warmed up, I'd take the garbage bag off. After all, I was pretty proud of being all the way from Hawaii. I also knew that I would probably get a lot of support from the hundreds of spectators who lined the marathon course. I was certainly going to need the interaction with and encouragement from the spectators to help me get through the 26.2 miles ahead in my apparently weakened condition.

At the 10-mile mark, I took off the gloves. Within minutes, my fingers got so numb that I couldn't hold the paper cups supplying liquid refreshment at the aid stations. I knew that I needed to drink a lot of water and stay hydrated. On went the gloves again. At the 20-mile mark, I was still cold. *This is ridiculous*, I thought. But what the heck! Since I was that cold, I figured that I had better keep the garbage bag on. In retrospect, I think it was the anemia that kept me from warming up.

Then I saw the official photographer taking pictures of all the runners. *Enough's enough*, I thought, and off came the garbage bag. I was not about to have an official photo show me running the Boston Marathon in a garbage bag. In the end, I finished in a halfway-decent time and was glad I'd persisted, gambled, and won. What an unforgettable experience and an exciting race! Afterwards, it took months of taking iron pills to get me back to normal. My low hemoglobin went back up first over a period of about three months, but it was nearly a year before my ferritin iron stores registered normal again.

This happened in 1984, when most medical personnel did not know a great deal about some of the maladies that could affect long-distance runners. The main lesson that I learned was to always monitor the color of my stools. Any bleeding from the GI tract causes darker stools. This would be immediately obvious if you're a vegan because a plant-based diet yields normally lighter-colored stools. In time, from reading medical journals, I would also learn that partaking in hard races and triathlons can cause several days of GI bleeding and that GI bleeding is common in long-distance runners, vegan or not.

Most physicians I have talked to seem to think that the bleeding comes from the stomach; Dr. Kent C. Holtzmuller, on the other hand, claims that it comes from the colon. He explains that the stomach has a double blood supply and is not as vulnerable to the effects of blood being shifted to the working muscles; meanwhile, the colon has a single blood supply and, as a result, suffers damage when there's an inadequate blood flow to its cells, which then die. According to Dr. Holtzmuller, almost all marathoners have traces of blood in their stools at the end of a race.[1]

Having found out the hard way that naproxen causes GI bleeding and that there are no anti-inflammatory drugs that will not do the same, I also became much more cautious about the use of NSAIDs—non-steroidal, anti-inflammatory drugs that are still commonly used for aches and pains—especially since they are heavily advertised and sold over the counter. NSAIDs are appropriate only for short-term treatment because two major possible side effects of long-term use are GI bleeding and liver damage. Thankfully, I rarely, if ever, need them anymore.

I wonder how many people have GI bleeding and don't know it. If you eat the SAD diet, filled with animal products, you'd have to bleed quite a lot to see black, tarry stools (consuming animal meat—and, by extension, animal blood—already yields dark stools). There is a test for occult bleeding that you should be able to get from your doctor to take at home. It's a good test to use to check for not only GI bleeding from racing but also colon cancer, which, unfortunately, is striking younger and younger folks now. The American Cancer Society recommends that people at average risk get this test done annually, starting at age forty-five. Of course, I believe that if you're eating a meat-centered diet, your risk is far more than average.

CHAPTER SEVENTEEN

LOOKING GOOD, FEELING SEXY

While walking to the start line of a 10K race one Saturday, I caught sight of Susan, a young elite (super-fast) runner. She, too, was walking to the start line. Alongside her was an obviously in-shape young man. Susan was talking away animatedly and reached out to give him a couple of pats on the behind. I smiled, broke into a little jog, and said as I passed her, "Keep your mind on the race, Susan!" All three of us had a good laugh and an excellent race. (We all won in our respective divisions.)

I cite this incident not only because I smile every time I think about it but also because it illustrates a point. Fitness is sexy. When you look around and see a sea of fit, trim bodies, that is sexy. And when you feel good about your body, it returns the favor. Whereas excess fat covers up your muscles, making your body less attractive, a lack thereof allows the same firm, curvy muscles to show through. This is true irrespective of your sex or age. We all have the same basic skeleton, the same basic musculature, and therefore the same potential for a beautiful body. Indeed, we are born quite similar to each other and only diversify as we age; we are the most different in old age, after a lifetime of being shaped by an interplay of genetics and lifestyle factors.

Sexiness starts with the initial, physical attractiveness of having a beautiful body. Then, when two people run together, they tend to open up and share their thoughts and concerns, many of them very intimate in nature. This creates a strong emotional bond, something you can experience even with people you have never seen before and may never see again. The bond is there. I can remember people I ran with ten years ago, especially if they were encouraging me at a time when I was sagging and needed it. It works the other way around too: there are people whom I have encouraged during a race who have thanked me years later.

Let's not forget the value system that fit people have in common. Athletes value their bodies, health, and performance, and they appreciate others who share these values. Conversely, athletes may find it difficult to enjoy people who abuse their bodies—whether it's by eating the wrong foods, getting unhealthy, smoking, using drugs and alcohol, or not exercising—or who just don't care.

These psychological aspects aside, a fit body simply functions better. A fit body has a stronger heart, wide-open arteries and capillaries, with blood that carries more nutrients—oxygen, minerals, antioxidants, and phytonutrients—to every cell.

Who Needs Viagra Anyway?

Some male runners have noticed that they have stronger erections when they get in better cardiovascular shape and especially when they change their diet.[1] This is very likely because as cardiovascular condition improves, the blood supply to the penis becomes more abundant. And since an erection is a vascular event, it is logical to assume that a better vascular condition increases the quality of erections. After all, erections are dependent on a good blood supply, and a good blood supply is the reward of both a low-fat, whole-food, plant-based diet and regular, vigorous exercise.

There seems to be a popularly accepted notion that as men age, their erections diminish in strength. The hoopla that greeted the introduction of Viagra and similar drugs is evidence that the modern Western lifestyle is causing erectile problems. Wouldn't you imagine that a man who has no trouble getting erect would have no need or interest in a drug like Viagra? The clogging of the tiny blood vessels that supply blood to the penis, not aging, explains why erectile dysfunction occurs—a process that leads to impotence if it continues unimpeded.

The smart man, who values the sensual side of life and is wary of the potential negative side effects of taking drugs, therefore has another good reason to eat a low-fat, whole-food vegan diet and get lots of vigorous exercise. This applies equally to women, whose reproductive system also needs an unrestricted blood supply (to the vagina, clitoris, uterus, and so on) to function, which is dependent on wide-open arteries and capillaries. Indeed, women can suffer from a form of "erectile dysfunction" themselves.

Keeping a Healthy Prostate

For men, another benefit of this program concerns prostate health. The prostate is a gland that surrounds the neck of the bladder and the urethra. As men in the West age, their prostates tend to enlarge, frequently to the point where their urine stream is greatly diminished, leading to a number of urinary-tract problems and even putting them at risk of prostate cancer. Indeed, most people, including physicians, think that this enlargement of the prostate (called benign prostatic hypertrophy) is inevitable with time. It is taken as a matter of fact that older men can't empty their bladders completely and, as a result, have to get up frequently during the night to urinate, thus disrupting a good night's sleep. (The medical term for frequent nighttime urination is nocturia.)

What's really interesting is that in countries whose populations eat a diet closer to a low-fat vegan diet and further from the SAD diet, men don't suffer from benign prostatic hypertrophy, and the incidence of prostate cancer is low.[2] As evidence shows, it's primarily the excess hormones in dairy and other animal products that overstimulate the prostate.

Estrogen and Progesterone

There is a great deal about women's hormones that is not widely known and a great deal that remains to be discovered. For example, the important role played by progesterone has been discovered only in the recent past.[3] For years, it was thought that women's estrogen levels were usually too low, and estrogen supplementation was prescribed to women regardless of their symptoms. If a woman complained of symptoms of premenstrual syndrome (PMS), she was put on estrogen when in reality, she was probably producing too much estrogen. Fibrocystic breasts, estrogen-positive breast cancer, fibroids, heavy menstrual bleeding, mood swings, weight gain, and bloating may all be indicative of estrogen dominance.

Estrogen exposure has increased radically in just a few generations. It has been estimated that before the Industrial Revolution, women had approximately 150 menstrual cycles, whereas modern women have 400 cycles. Children consuming the SAD diet are subject to precocious sexual maturity, with girls starting their periods from the age of eight or nine instead of sixteen or seventeen as it used to be. An earlier onset of menstruation aside, fewer pregnancies, lower lactation rates, shorter lactation periods, and a later menopause all contribute to a higher number of cycles in a woman's lifetime. This increased exposure to estrogen thus leads to all the symptoms mentioned above.

Estrogen levels only *appear* to drop abruptly with the onset of menopause. A woman's estrogen actually begins dropping around the age of thirty-five, which is when some doctors begin recommending estrogen supplements, assumed to prevent heart disease and bone loss. However, if she eats a low-fat, plant-based vegan diet and gets lots of exercise, her risk of heart disease drops and she will have no problem maintaining her bone mass. Many women on the SAD diet actually have very high levels of estrogen, high enough that they suffer the symptoms of estrogen dominance and an increased risk of breast cancer. The last thing these women need is more estrogen!

In addition to a good diet and exercise regime, what might help women is natural progesterone to balance their estrogen. (Natural progesterone is different from the progesterone in the pharmaceutical drug progestin; many, even health professionals I've spoken to, confuse the two.) Since most progesterone is produced during ovulation, we know that when a woman reaches menopause, she will be deficient in progesterone. Fortunately, this can be easily remedied with supplementation from a plant source of progesterone, usually soy or the Mexican wild yam (*Dioscorea*).[4] This supplement product frequently takes the form of a cream (trans-dermal) because when the hormone goes through the skin, it avoids a first pass through the liver. This is important because one of the liver's jobs is to clear hormones from the blood. Progesterone has also been shown to reverse osteoporosis and maintain libido in women.[5] Possible applications of trans-dermal progesterone in shrinking the prostate and stopping the growth of prostate cancer in men are also being explored.[6]

Women with symptoms of low estrogen may be prescribed a form of horse estrogen in the drug Premarin, derived from pregnant mares' urine. The poor mares are forced to stand still, never being able to move, so that all of the urine during their pregnancy can be collected in bags, usually for nine months. This terrible cruelty notwithstanding, horse estrogen is not quite comparable to human estrogen, and the use of horse estrogen brings with it many unwanted side effects, not least of which is an increased risk of breast cancer. By contrast, progesterone has been discovered to normalize cancerous and other abnormal breast cells subject to excess stimulation by estrogen.[7]

The "female" hormones play at least a partial role in many functions of a woman's body, including the development and maintenance of feminine characteristics (e.g., breasts, soft skin, a higher-pitched voice), hair-growth rates and patterns, vaginal health, bone strength, healing, and so on. As it turns out, diet has a significant influence on estrogen levels: without the overstimulation of animal protein, vegan women have normal estrogen levels; they also excrete more estrogen in their stools than do omnivorous women and produce twice the fecal bulk. Even urinary levels of estrogen are lower in vegan women, which, since estrogen is easily re-absorbed through the intestinal walls, leave less estrogen available for re-absorption and ultimately contribute to lowering the risk of breast cancer.[8]

Because men are also subject to some of the diseases thought to be limited to women, I will point out that about 1 percent of breast cancer cases are in men. I will never forget the day that I met Lou P. Knowing who I was, he excitedly shared, "We have more in common than you think!" With that, he pulled open his shirt, exposing a long, horizontal scar—a souvenir from a modified radical mastectomy. So guys, remember that breast self-exam is for everybody!

The Fountain of Youth?
There are so many good reasons for both men and women to take good care of themselves, but probably the most sensual aspect of fitness is the glowing vitality that a fit person exudes. That, to me, is the sexiest of all!

Vitality is no respecter of age, and fitness seems to put a hold on—if not, in some instances, reverse—the aging process. There are a number of ways to measure the body's biological age, among them strength, speed, flexibility, endurance, blood pressure, resting heart rate, body-fat percentage, cholesterol level, ability to process oxygen, and telomere length. Strenuous exercise, along with a low-fat, high-complex-carbohydrate diet, affects every one of these measures. It is the closest thing you'll ever find to a "fountain of youth"!

A sad fact is that as people get older, they tend to put on more body fat—even if they don't gain a pound—because they lose muscle and bone, a condition called sarcopenia. This is not sexy, right? Bodies that are lean, muscular, and taut are attractive at any age. One way to fight increasing body fat is to increase exercise. A way for you to make exercise fun is to do it with friends. Another way to keep you motivated to stay active is to enter races. Races are also a lot of fun, which is why people keep coming back.

You'd best believe that glowing good health will also do wonders for your sex drive. When you feel good about yourself and your body, a natural sex appeal just exudes from your pores. You are attractive to other people, and you'll probably find yourself turned on by other people who are sexy and fit. Wouldn't you like to have a healthy, active sex life until you're in your eighties and nineties, and—who knows—possibly even beyond?

The old saying "use it or lose it" definitely applies here. As women pass menopause, they experience symptoms such as a thinning of the vaginal walls and a lack of lubrication. According to some authorities, the best treatment is continued and frequent usage. Indeed, gynecologists can usually tell if older women are not sexually active by the shrinkage of the vagina and the thinning of its walls. In the book *How a Woman Ages*, science writer Robin Marantz Henig even makes the claim that women should remain sexually active all their lives, even if they have to accomplish this themselves, to keep their vaginal tissue healthy.[9]

By the way, here's a bit of information that I find absolutely amazing. I was once told by a veterinarian that humans are the only species whose females undergo menopause. All other female mammals maintain an estrus cycle, meaning that their ovaries keep producing sex hormones and their sexual activity continues, for the duration of their natural lives.

Too Pooped to Pop?

You may have heard that vigorous exercise leads to a diminished sex drive. This is probably the case for those in the initial phases of their training program, who are experiencing adjustments as they begin to increase their training. The condition is soon reversed as their bodies adapt to being under heavier stress.

While anything can certainly be taken to an unhealthy extreme, this does not happen very often in the case of exercise. The greater risk lies in doing too little, not too much. By way of illustration, ask yourself how many people you have heard of who over-exercise. Now ask yourself how many people you know who do little or no exercise. Most of the people I know are relatively sedentary and not at any risk of doing too much. Indeed, I've never met anyone who exercises too much.

Swimming Is Sexy!

A study reported in *Swim Magazine* found that middle-aged and older men and women committed to regular swim workouts had sex lives that were as active as those of people in their late twenties and early thirties.[10] Furthermore, as long as they maintained their fitness program, their libido and sexual activity did not decline with age. Swimmers in their sixties were as active as non-swimmers in their forties. And not only were the swimmers more active sexually, they also enjoyed sex more, according to the rating scale used. This makes sense because love-making is a physical act in which strength, agility, and endurance count. The weak, tired, and out-of-shape person cannot hold up very well or very long. By contrast, strong, energetic, and fit lovers can throw themselves enthusiastically into love-making and last a lot longer. Yes, fit people of any age make better lovers.

Unfortunately, among Americans, there is a notion that sex is an activity largely reserved for the young and beautiful. With many of our sex symbols being in their late teens and early twenties, the idea of the elderly engaging in sexual activity is foreign to most people—and foreign to older people themselves if they are in poor physical condition or are embarrassed about their bodies.

The opposite reality is possible. We can have older people who are still physically vigorous, who feel good about their strong, supple bodies. They have the energy and desire to continue leading active sex lives for as long as they want. And it appears that being in superb physical condition would make them want to be active. This is probably because sex drive is dependent on the so-called "male" sex hormone, testosterone (I say "so-called" because testosterone is present in women as well, though in lesser quantities). Studies have shown that physical activity increases levels of testosterone in both men and women while decreasing levels of the so-called "female" hormone, estrogen (again, I say "so-called" because men also produce estrogen, though less of it). (Hence also why women who train excessively may stop having their periods.)

In true cases of over-exercise, sex drive in both sexes can suffer, likely due to fatigue and a reduced availability of time. It will bounce back quickly, however, once the excessive training stops. This resurgence is probably accelerated by the fact that athletes tend to have an improved self-image: they look and feel younger and more beautiful.

Beauty Tips for Athletes

Many people falsely perceive women athletes as jocks (or "jockettes"). Accompanying this misperception is the implication that being athletic is the antithesis of being feminine—that "beautiful competitor" is an oxymoron. As I got more and more into hard training and competing, I was faced with the inevitable conflicts. *If I do a swim workout, my hair will be ruined; and I may as well forget about make-up. If I put on a bicycle helmet, I'll also end up with a flattened, sweaty head of hair.* And who can present a decent face when they're dripping with perspiration?

There was another conflict. On race day, I usually had to get up way before the crack of dawn, sometimes three or four o'clock in the morning. Who could possibly be thinking of looking gorgeous at a time like that, especially when their mind needs to be on the race? Not willing to give up all vestiges of attractiveness, I developed a bunch of beauty tricks. Some of them are very practical and some purely frivolous. I would not give up any of them. See if there is a trick that suits you.

Permanent eyeliner and brows. If applied correctly, this procedure is done once and forgotten about forever. You wake up with beautiful eyes and brows; you come out of the water with beautiful eyes and brows; you cross the finish line with beautiful eyes and brows. I've had my permanent eyeliner and brows long enough that I "own" them. They are so much part of me that I forget I ever really needed them.

With the liner and brows, I get by without any make-up. This really paid off when the reporters from the *New Zealand Herald* took photos of me, including a close-up, right after I crossed the finish line of the Ironman. My picture on the front page of the newspaper showed eyes that could have just stepped out of a make-up artist's studio—well, almost!

Dealing with presbyopia. When I reached the age of forty-seven, I finally had to face the fact that reading small print was becoming impossible. As I looked around, I saw people approaching forty who were having to convert to bifocal glasses. I had thought that maybe I'd escape that fate, but no, I had just been lucky in being able to put it off for a bit. When I mentioned to my boss that I was going to have to see an eye doctor, he revealed to me his "secret": he wore contact lenses with one side set for close-up reading and the other for distance vision (monovision).

Since my distance vision was fine, I asked an optometrist if I could wear just one lens. He didn't see any reason why I couldn't. I asked if he had any other patient who did that, and he told me that I would be his first (we're talking about the late 1970s). Well, this was a little scary, but I figured I didn't have much to lose. Monovision worked like a charm. For years, I was able to avoid eyeglasses. After swimming, I came out of the water able to see everything. If I had a bike problem, I could see close-up details to fix it. And after a race, I could read the posted results, which was helpful since I frequently covered race events as a reporter. Then, when LASIK (laser-assisted in situ keratomileusis) surgery became available as a permanent solution to far-sightedness, I made the jump and had my "reading eye" corrected, which gave me the same vision without contact lenses. The freedom was wonderful.

I'm willing to bet that you, too, want eyes that stay healthy and functional for as long as possible. Yet again, diet plays an important role. Studies show that those who eat the most leafy greens have the lowest risk of cataracts and glaucoma.[11] Furthermore, a whole-food, plant-based diet helps prevent age-related macular degeneration, the most common cause of blindness in people over sixty-five.[12]

Hair and skin. I've had my hair short; I've had it down to my waist. Either way works for me, but short hair is certainly a lot easier to stuff under a swim cap or a helmet, or to shampoo after each one of multitudinous workouts. There is probably only one prerequisite, and that is to have a simple hairstyle. Then, when you cross the finish line of a race, all you have to do is run a comb through your hair. You'll look perfectly groomed and ready for the cameras, since you'll surely want some photos of your "triathletic" accomplishments. Plus, when you exude good health, you don't need to rely on a fancy hairdo to make you beautiful!

Taking care of your skin is important as well. When your blood is healthy—packed with oxygen and nutrients from your good diet—and your circulation top-notch, your skin positively glows, which pretty much eliminates the need for any kind of make-up.

Do use sunblock, however; sweat and salt water will not harm your skin, but too much sun will. There is no quicker way to age your skin than with too much exposure to the sun. Since it's a little difficult to get your training done in the dark, the only solution is to use as close to a total sunblock as possible when you go on a long run or bike ride in the midday sun. There are now sunblocks on the market with a sun protection factor (SPF) of 50 or more. This means that if you normally get sunburned after one minute, wearing sunblock will in theory give you fifty or more minutes before you start to get burned. Since some sunblocks contain chemicals that you don't want, you can also use zinc oxide, which acts as a mechanical, no-chemical block. Dermatologists will tell you that sunblock application should be an automatic ritual before going outside during the day. Indeed, it'll pay off as you get older!

Sunglasses. The sun can damage not only your skin but also your eyes, causing cataracts to form. This is where sunglasses come in handy. Just make sure the lenses are coated with a filter to screen out ultraviolet rays. Sunglasses also tend to minimize the lines in the outer corner of the eyes (endearingly called "laugh lines") formed over time from repeated frowning and squinting, both of which also lead to facial wrinkles.

Legs. I'm sure you've seen women, some of them quite young, who have unsightly spider veins or even large, knotty varicose veins in their legs. These are not entirely reversible, although it's possible to prevent them or stop their progression by eating a high-fiber diet (which is what a whole-food, plant-based diet is) and getting lots of good circulation in the legs through activities such as running and biking.

Varicose veins are caused by the failure of the venous valves to stop the backflow of blood as it journeys from the feet up to the heart. As you can imagine, there's a lot of pressure from that blood trying to go upstream against gravity, and incompetent valves will let the blood pool in the veins, leading to tortuous twisted, knotted veins. Not only is this unattractive, but blood clots can form in the stagnating blood that can break free, and if one gets to the lungs, it can cause a potentially fatal pulmonary embolism.

A lot of people think that their varicose veins are hereditary, saying that this condition runs in their family. Sure, you tend to have the same kind of valves your parents do. But guess what is also usually inherited? Dietary habits. And while there is nothing you can do about your genes, you have a lot of power to improve the health of your veins with the help of a whole-food, plant-based vegan diet.

Consider this: People who don't get enough fiber in their diets have bowel problems such as constipation. (If you have reading material in your bathroom, you're probably not getting enough fiber!) Constipation causes straining, which puts tremendous pressure on the veins in the lower half of the body. Constipated people raise their risk of getting not only varicose veins in their legs but also hemorrhoids. In addition to not enough fiber in the diet, a sedentary lifestyle contributes to varicose veins, constipation, hemorrhoids, and possibly even prolapse of the bowel. So here's another important reason to exercise.

Feet. With proper-fitting shoes, or preferably no shoes (it is nature's way, after all), we should all have beautiful feet. Unfortunately, this is not the case. Runners can have black toenails from running downhill in shoes that are too short, thickened toenails from hitting their toes against the ends of shoes with a toe box that is too small, and blisters from rubbing on areas where there is friction. These are usually temporary conditions that one can relieve by getting rid of the offending shoes.

Feet expand with usage, and most people find that their feet grow one or two sizes when they take up running. Therefore, you need to be sure to get shoes in a size large enough to accommodate the spreading of the foundation for your body. Feet also tend to expand from morning to evening, so buy shoes later in the day. Bike shoes, on the other hand, are fitted differently. They need to be very snug as your body's forces are transmitted through them directly to the pedals, and you will probably need to do little, if any, walking in them.

If you tend to develop calluses on the bottom of your feet, take every opportunity you can to walk barefoot in the sand. Not only will this strengthen your foot muscles, it will also grind off your calluses, leaving baby-smooth skin.

Beauty Tips from Magazines and Books

Personally, I think many of the diet and beauty tips given in the latest magazines and celebrity-authored books count as false advertising, intended only to make money by taking advantage of the desire of a majority of people to be more attractive. We now know that much of this advice can even be harmful.

For example, we now know that the much-hyped high-protein and liquid-protein diets, often full of animal products, can damage bones and kidneys. Within hours of any animal protein being consumed, the kidneys have to rev up into hyper-filtration mode, which can eventually cause irreversible kidney damage. This explains why there are so many kidney dialysis centers popping up all over. You definitely want to avoid kidney failure as it requires radical changes to your lifestyle and the prognosis is not good, usually with a life expectancy of five years or less.[13] By contrast, the plant protein from a whole-food, plant-based diet can save your kidneys.

Then you may read about low-calorie diets. These will just put your body in a semi-starvation mode in which you lose not only fat but also muscle. You'll probably feel too weak to get any exercise, and the muscles that you don't use will start to atrophy very quickly, becoming weak and slack. When the deprivation period is over and you overcompensate for it, which, of course, is inevitable, you'll also end up with more body fat than before as your body learns to stock up in case of scarcity. Bones that don't get put under stress regularly suffer the same fate of atrophy and weakness. Indeed, sexy curves are from muscle-toning exercise, not from caloric restriction, liposuction, or silicone.

You don't need make-up to make your skin glow. Your "rouge" is the natural color of the vasomotor flush from strenuous exercise. Your "foundation" is the soft, fine-pored skin that is the result of good nutrients supplied to the epithelial cells by a strong circulatory system. Lipstick is unnecessary when your lips are healthy and pink from the underlying bright-red blood. Likewise, your teeth look whiter when your gums are a healthy, deeper pink from a bountiful blood supply. And don't forget to, at least once a day, floss the teeth you'd like to keep (that is, all of them, presumably). All the exercise in the world cannot get rid of the plaque that develops around your gum lines and that can cause periodontal disease and the loss of even healthy teeth. Finally, bright, sexy eyes are the result of your getting an adequate amount of deep sleep each night after being physically and mentally active all day long, plus your enthusiasm for life and living when you treat your body as it should be treated—as all bodies would be treated if we only came with a perfect "owner's manual."

So forget about artificial beauty tricks. When you're in doubt about whether or not to try something, ask the question: is it natural? Now, if it isn't, that doesn't automatically mean that you shouldn't do it. You just have to know what you are doing and evaluate the risk versus the benefit. All I'm offering here is a way for you to make healthy living a lot of fun and a lifelong commitment. I know that once you try this lifestyle, you'll never go back to your old ways—ever. When you are at your healthiest, you will automatically be at your most attractive—and you can remain so for the rest of your life.

What Alcohol Does to Your Body

Now, a word about alcohol and its effects on your body. First of all, you should know that alcohol is toxic to all living cells. Its effects on the body's systems are so scary that you'd think if people only knew, they'd stay as far away from it as possible.

Because alcohol is a solvent, it gets to every cell in your body, subsequently changing the biochemical functions inside the cell. Alcohol, like other drugs, can plug into the receptor sites on the surface of the cell membrane, causing "desirable" sensations such as intoxication. (Notice *toxic* in the middle of the word.) It causes changes in the bilipid (fat) layers of the cell, although there is less damage if you are on a low-fat diet. And it wreaks general havoc on cell-receptor function, even destroying receptors.

Your liver performs more than four hundred different functions, one of which is to detoxify poisons such as the alcohol in beer, sake, and bourbon. Unfortunately, chronic use of alcohol knocks off liver cells. Liver enzymes then start leaking into the bloodstream. Continued exposure to alcohol leads to hepatitis and cirrhosis (scarring). The poor, besieged liver contracts, which causes an increase in blood pressure, and becomes hampered in its ability to break down estrogen. This leads to the development of gynecomastia, or "man boobs."

If you're a woman, the increase of estrogen heightens your risk of breast cancer, which is bad enough. If, however, you're a man, this is also really bad news for your sex life. Your testicles will start to shrivel and breast tissue will start to form. In fact, gynecomastia is a telltale sign that physicians look for in checking for alcoholism. Eventually, men become impotent while women also suffer impaired fertility, and both can experience a loss of libido (sex drive) and become anorgasmic (unable to have an orgasm).[14] If you value your sexuality, you sure have enough reasons to stay away from alcohol.

So you see, there's a lot more to glowing good health than most people realize. For several reasons, fitness is sexy, and if you're fit enough to do triathlons, you're probably in top sexual form as well. Now you know what triathletes are referring to when they talk about the fourth event!

Chapter Eighteen

Killer Breasts: Reconstruction and Breast Implant Illness

Since it was my cancerous breasts that were trying to kill me, I was more than ready to get rid of them. Amid those harrowing days of dealing with my diagnosis and getting ready for the mastectomy, there appeared a small ray of sunshine. I had remembered reading about reconstructive surgery and asked my surgeon about it. He said he'd arrange for me to have a consultation with the plastic surgery department.

One of the books I'd read said that there was a "quaint" theory that some plastic surgeons still held regarding breast reconstruction. They were recommending that breast reconstruction be withheld from patients for approximately two years, thinking that if a woman had to do without breasts for at least that period of time, when the reconstruction was accomplished, she'd be grateful for whatever she had gotten. It seems that the technology was not that great back in 1982, and in fact, some of the least successful results bordered on the grotesque. By the way, this has all changed; these days, in most cases, reconstruction is done simultaneous to the mastectomy.

I had expected to see the plastic surgeon before my mastectomy but was told that he was "too busy." Dismayed, I recalled another book that suggested that the plastic surgeon should participate in the surgical procedure of the mastectomy itself to ensure that nothing would be done to complicate the later surgery. I had no choice then but to take my chances. As it turned out, the book was right.

When I finally saw the plastic surgeon, about two months after my surgery, he shook his head at the location of my two scars from drainage tubes that had been put almost in the middle of where my new breasts would sit. It was too bad that they had been placed there, he said; the resultant scar tissue had made his job a lot harder. I saw nothing to gain by protesting and just heaved a big sigh.

Nonetheless, after examining me, the plastic surgeon told me that I was an excellent candidate for reconstruction. Elated, I asked how soon I could have the operation. "As soon as the scar softens and the skin stretches enough to take the implant," he said. In a mastectomy, in an effort to eliminate all possible vagrant cancer cells lying underneath the skin and in the subcutaneous fat, surgeons cut away as much skin as possible and scrape the subcutaneous fat from the "flaps" they create to cover the now-bare rib cage and close the wound. My procedure was no exception. As a result, my chest now looked flatter than a pre-pubescent child's, and my ribs stuck out. It was difficult to move my arms in any direction because my skin had been stretched so tightly to cover the chest wall.

What my plastic surgeon and I did not discuss was the possibility of using my own tissue to form a breast mound, such as with a latissimus dorsi flap (muscle surgically brought around from the back) or tissue from a "tummy tuck" (tissue moved upwards from the stomach). The plan he had for me was to insert silicone implants, which, at the time, seemed the simplest and by far least invasive answer.

What I Didn't Know I Didn't Know

What I did not know at the time were the questions that I should have asked: Where was the evidence that silicone implants are safe? Would they last a lifetime or have to be exchanged periodically, meaning more surgeries? Would the implants be inserted just under the skin or under the pectoralis, the chest muscle? What are the pros and cons of each method? Does the under-the-muscle placement require cutting and moving parts of muscles to make room for the implants? Would that not affect the strength and length of my swim stroke? Since we know that scar tissue does not stretch, would the scars make me feel like I'm in an "iron bra"? Would this keep me from taking a full, deep breath (yes, it would!)?

I simply agreed to what I was told, making an unwarranted assumption that of course, my surgeon would do whatever procedure was best for me, that the silicone implants were safe—or he wouldn't be using them. I knew absolutely nothing then about how the body's immune system would immediately identify breast implants as foreign bodies and would start trying to attack them just as it would viruses, bacteria, and fungi. Since implants don't die like the latter do, there would be a constant war, which sets up a low-grade, chronic inflammation. I have to assume now that my plastic surgeon didn't know that either.

He told me that it would take a minimum of six months to a year for my scars to soften and my skin to stretch. Indeed, he said, it might never happen, in which case they would resort to skin grafts, a prospect I did not relish at all. I was very conscientious about doing frequent stretching exercises and even pulling on the skin for good measure. It must have worked because during my third visit at four months, the surgeon told me that I had made good progress. My surgery was scheduled for two months later.

Looking back, I don't know how I got through those days. Every shower, every swim, every glance in the mirror was a stark reminder of not only my breastless form but also the cancer. Stuffing my bras with prostheses just did not do the trick. Every time I raised my arm, the whole bra slid up. When I lowered my arm, the bra and prostheses stayed up. I remember one day, during a swim, I saw one of my prostheses floating away! What an uncomfortable, miserable way to live. I felt like I was holding my breath until the day of the surgery.

The day I was admitted to the hospital, I had to go through all the usual pre-op tests. For the first time, I did so with great excitement and enthusiasm. I grinned at the lab tech as she drew my blood. I babbled on as the electrocardiogram technician checked the condition of my heart, telling her that this was the last time electrodes were placed on this chicken-breasted form. She paid no attention to me as she seemed to be having trouble with the machine. I asked if something was wrong. She turned to me, "Are you a *runner?*"

"Yes, why?"

"That explains it," she said. "I was getting a heart rate of 44!" Since the average adult's heart rate is about 72, this put me in the extremely fit category. She said she had never seen a woman with a heart rate that low.

Next, the plastic surgeon took his purple marker and drew all sorts of marks on me: a nipple line across my chest so that my nipples would be even post-reconstruction, two circles for the areolas (the pigmented areas around the nipples), two lower lines for the inframammary folds (medical speak for the lower curves of my new breasts), as well as marks on my ears and thighs. My earlobes were to contribute a wedge of skin and cartilage, to be sculpted into two nipples, and my upper inner thighs were to donate the skin for two new areolas.

"Just the right hint of pink too," the plastic surgeon joked.

That night in the hospital, I could hardly sleep. The plastic surgeon had impressed on me that the choices I had made as to the exact size and location of my new breasts were irreversible. I'd better be sure, he had said. I got up several times during the night to check myself in the mirror. Were they going to be too big? Too small? Too high? Too low? Too far apart? Too close together?

Wait a minute, I thought. *What did my old breasts use to look like?* I couldn't remember! I thought then that maybe those surgeons who insisted on delaying reconstruction surgery had the right idea—make them wait and they'll be grateful for anything. And I was grateful for my new breasts—for a while. The healing seemed to go very well for the first month. Then, one day, I noticed that one "breast" was higher than the other. Or was it that the other one was too low? Over the period of a couple of months, it seemed to be getting worse. I returned for a check-up and remarked on the discrepancy.

The plastic surgeon brushed off my concern, reasoning that nothing on the body that is paired is identical—that one's feet are two different sizes, one's legs are two different lengths, and so on. I told him that while I agreed to a point, the discrepancy I was experiencing had passed that point: I felt like a ship whose cargo had shifted and which was "listing" to one side. Finally, when he realized I was not going to be mollified, he agreed to a correction.

By this time, I was an old hand at surgery, and the thought of another operation didn't bother me in the least. It is a process, much like a marathon. You've got to go through a lot of discomfort sometimes to get what you want—to cross the finish line—but it would be worth it in the end. My new breasts became so much a part of me and my body image that I'd forgotten what I used to look like. And the best news of all, I thought, was that as I grew older, they would never sag. I chuckled to myself as I conjured up the image of a ninety-year-old triathlete with these nice, high, firm, round bosoms!

For the next thirty years, I felt "normal"—my days of being completely flat were long gone. I loved and proudly showed off my "killer breasts"!

Killer Breasts: Deconstruction and the Big Lie

It had been thirty years since the damning diagnosis, and the threat of the breast cancer recurring had diminished significantly. I was rolling along with everything, finally seeming to be good with life. I had known that I was getting "old" when I had turned seventy, but I was feeling no signs of aging, no loss of energy, or anything other than a carefree sense that getting older is no big deal. At this point, I had been a runner for almost forty years. At seventy-one, I had written a second book published by Lantern, *Senior Fitness*. And when my editor, Martin Rowe (who had been inspired to give running a try after editing the manuscript of the first edition of this book and ended up running a number of marathons), asked me to write yet another book, this time about lifelong running, after much mulling over, I agreed, wanting to share the many benefits of being a dedicated runner with others. (The result was my third Lantern book, *Lifelong Running: Overcome the 11 Myths about Running and Live a Healthier Life*.)

My clock was ticking and I had absolutely no idea what was about to occur. For several years, microparticles of silicone and heavy metals from the silicone implants had been slowly leaching into my body for several years; the condition had started to reach an extremely critical threshold, at which the symptoms would become too obvious to ignore or rationalize away as I had been doing.

Ominous Signs: What Was Coming Next

Back in 2010, I started noticing that while walking, I had the feeling like I was on a ship and the experience of "sea legs" as I compensated for this loss of balance. I started dropping things and kept bumping into doorways, which indicated a loss of proprioception (a sense of where I was in space). I reported this to my doctor to ask what could be the cause. He said that he didn't know and simply wrote a prescription for a seasickness drug that he said should help. Well, it didn't at all, but he had nothing else to offer. He said that I was just going to have to live with it and hope that it'd eventually go away. On the contrary, my balance kept getting worse.

Next, I noticed that my feet felt like they were enclosed in tight-fitting gloves, with a sensation of a cool breeze blowing through. This was especially noticeable when I was swimming. When I was wearing running shoes and socks, I was puzzled by just the cool breeze: it made sense that I felt like my feet were enclosed because of the shoes, but the mystery remained as to why there was a breeze, even in Hawaii's warm tropical weather.

Several years later, I went back to my doctor, trying again to find out what was causing all of these weird symptoms. He ordered a bunch of blood tests, reviewed the results that all came back normal, and again said that he had no answers, but this time, I was not ready to give up. Thus began a round of visits to specialists, starting with a neurologist since I felt my impaired balance was putting me at dangerously high risk of falling.

The first test was to see if I had benign paroxysmal positional vertigo (BPPV), a condition of the inner ear in which tiny calcium carbonate crystals called canaliths or otoliths get displaced, which can cause feelings of imbalance. I didn't have that, so I was referred to a balance therapist and given a series of exercises to do. These might have helped a little, but my balance was still poor. Up to that point, I had fallen three times; each time, I had fallen backwards, luckily landing on my rear end and incurring no broken bones. Unfortunately, that was about to change.

In 2003, I started having fractures. The first occurred when I apparently tripped over something while running and fell. I had enough pain in my right arm to be alarmed and headed to the hospital. X-rays confirmed that it was a fracture of the upper-arm bone, the humerus. Later, I checked back to see what had tripped me up, but I had been on a smooth sidewalk. It was puzzling indeed, especially since the same sequence of events happened again in 2014, this time resulting in a fracture of a lower-arm bone, the radius, in my left arm.

I then had a series of four rib fractures that involved not falls but just ordinary activities—bending over to put on a sock, turning over in bed, hoisting myself out of a pool, and receiving a big hug from the back. I knew that my previous bone scans in the early 1990s had shown very high-density bones. Since it had been several years since I'd had any bone-density measurement taken, in 2019, I took another test. The result this time was a minus 3.5, indicating severe osteoporosis. I was shocked! I had been doing everything right to keep my bones strong—keeping to the right diet and the right exercise. Doctors attributed this decline in bone density to aging and loss of estrogen. Since my cancer was estrogen-positive, they ruled out estrogen-replacement therapy. My only choice was to be put on a bone-building drug, which, if you remember from the chapter on osteoporosis, doesn't actually build bone. Knowing that the drug would have severe side effects, I thought that surely, if I kept up my healthy routine, my condition should get better.

The scan in 2021 gave me a bone-density measurement that was not only not better but even worse, a minus 3.7. I'd thought that a minus 3.5 was as bad as it could get! This time, the doctors really pushed for the drug. Again, I hesitantly looked at the side effects, some of which I could see that I was already having, including random joint pains, heart palpitations, chronic fatigue, and balance issues. I did not think I could handle these symptoms getting worse. The doctors then said that since it had been more than thirty years with no recurrence of my cancer, it was worth taking a risk and trying estrogen-replacement therapy to see if it would help increase my bone density. Knowing of no alternative, I chose the more natural course, which was to start estrogen replacement.

In the meantime, I started experiencing periodic joint pains in my left shoulder, right elbow, left wrist, fingers, both my upper and lower back, and—worst of all—my right knee. The pain was affecting my running and gradually got so bad that I had to seek out a physiatrist for help. Sure enough, x-rays and MRIs showed damage to the lateral meniscus in my right knee. He gave me hyaluronic acid injections, which helped for several months, but the pain came back. We then tried platelet-rich plasma (PRP) injections along with an eight-week course of physical therapy to strengthen the muscles supporting my knee. Stem cell injections, the most extreme method to heal a badly degenerated meniscus, also helped only temporarily.

At this point, it was getting increasingly painful to run. The situation got so bad that I was told that I was doing more damage to my knees if I continued to run. It soon got to the point at which it was painful just to walk.

I consulted Dr. Marumoto, the same orthopedic surgeon who'd put the tibial rod in my left leg back in 1998, who looked at the x-rays and said that I was definitely a candidate for a total knee replacement on my right leg.

Depressed, I mulled over the awful prospect. If I wanted to keep living independently, the choice was clear. When Dr. Marumoto told me that because I was so lean, I could even get back to running after surgery, I looked at all the alternatives one last time, swallowed real hard, and scheduled the surgery for two weeks later. Then, while doing one of the physical-therapy exercises that I'd been given, the "bridge," I suffered a compression fracture of the T12 thoracic vertebra. Naturally, this required a postponement of the knee replacement. I finally had my total knee replacement surgery in November 2019. With continued physical therapy, whole-body vibration, and aqua-jogging, I'm hoping that my left knee will be okay and that I may get back to "real" running. I still have goals to set to represent all of us seniors!

Then, alarmingly, short-term memory problems were added to the list of symptoms of my mystery illness; I started to have trouble finding words and names—to have so-called "brain fog." I was baffled by all of my symptoms, none of which I should be having, especially as there was no obvious cause. I had a normal blood pressure, normal cholesterol, normal A1C, and normal BMI—every test I was given returned normal results except for my low bone density and the joint damage in my knee, which I knew were not due to my running. If anything, we now know that running actually keeps the knees stronger, as I talked about earlier.

I'd consulted with fifteen different specialists and not one of them could offer any explanation except that it was just my age. I knew full well that it was not aging that was causing all of my symptoms. Patricia Blanchette, MD, a geriatrician at the University of Hawaii's John A. Burns School of Medicine who studies "really old people" and whom I love to quote, says that every symptom she has seen that has been attributed to age can be tied to either *disease* or *disuse*, joking that if someone is younger than eighty, she sends them back to their pediatrician. When I first heard that, two light bulbs went off in my head. *A-ha! Diet and exercise!* Almost all disease is due to an improper diet and disuse is atrophy from lack of exercise. I also kept recalling all the oldsters in the Blue Zones. I ruled out aging as the cause.

The other common suggestion was that I was just stressed out. Yes, I was stressed over all of these symptoms, but the stress was the *result* of the symptoms, hardly the cause. I even started having nightmares with scary episodes, including one in which I felt a coconut fall on my head. It was so real that I jumped and screamed out loud. Another night, I heard a loud voice announcing, "This is your last call!" I jumped out of bed so quickly that I tripped and nearly fell over some furniture as I tried to get to the phone. Of course, all I got was a dial tone. In an attempt to deal with the stress and stay rational, I started meditating daily and practicing mindfulness.

When the specialists finally gave up, unable to come up with any plausible cause, the verdict was "etiology unknown," the last resort. And yet, my symptoms went on, and the list seemed endless: chronic fatigue; insomnia; a chronic, productive cough; arrhythmias (irregular heart rhythms including supraventricular tachycardia); gastrointestinal upsets; alternating constipation and diarrhea; extreme nocturia (nighttime urination), with a need to urinate every hour for a total of two liters, the typical amount of liquid drunk in twenty-four hours; osteoporosis; joint pains; dry mouth and eyes; unexplained weight loss of thirty-five pounds; loss of balance; loss of proprioception; random, sharp, stabbing pains; weird muscle spasms that last up to two hours; major hair loss; and short-term memory problems. I realized that this whole series of symptoms had to add up to some specific cause. I knew that something was drastically wrong but could not figure out what it was, and neither could a single one of the many specialists I'd consulted.

My Living Nightmare Explained

On April 12, 2019, I picked up the morning newspaper and opened it up to see this headline: "Breast-Implant Illness a Nightmare." Having never heard of such a thing, I immediately dismissed the notion as ridiculous. At the time, I had had my breast implants for thirty-five years and still thought they were the perfect solution to my having had both my breasts chopped off. I was curious, though, and thought I might as well read the article to see what it had to say. As I read down the list of symptoms of "breast-implant illness," it hit me like a proverbial ton of bricks! I got weak in the knees as what I'd read hit home. It *had* to be my breast implants!

Where's the Evidence?

Just weeks before, on March 25, 2019, Jan Cohen Tervaert, MD, PhD, a rheumatologist at the University of Alberta in Edmonton, Canada, flew down to Washington, DC, on his own dime to brief the USDA on how, contrary to what had been previously thought, silicone breast implants are *not* inert but have a high risk of causing a range of autoimmune diseases. Dr. Tervaert made the case that the USDA must therefore *recall* and *ban* silicone breast implants.[1] His presentation revealed that there are micro-gel leaks from such implants that migrate to every part of the body and cause a wide range of symptoms such as joint pain, fever, sicca (dry mouth and eyes), cognitive impairment, lymphoma, and more.

Heavy-Metal Damage

Further, it was discovered that the danger lies in not just the silicone in the micro-gel, which bleeds directly into the body's circulatory system, but also the heavy metals that are used in the manufacture of implants. Indeed, lead, mercury, arsenic, cadmium, tin, zinc, platinum, aluminum, and other heavy metals can cross the protective blood–brain barrier and cause brain damage. In addition, they can disrupt metabolic function and damage the kidneys, liver, and central nervous system.[2]

The heavy metals penetrate each cell in the body all the way down to the microscopic level of the mitochondria—the little energy factories of the cell—poisoning the enzymes that transport nutrients to the mitochondria.[3] Mitochondria are key targets of the toxicity induced by heavy metals given their key role in the production of the body's energy, which explains my devastating chronic fatigue. As the brain consumes a large amount of energy, any dysfunction of the mitochondria may seriously disrupt brain function, which results in neuron death and neurological disorders. This explains my brain fog and balance issues.

Research has shown that lead has an affinity for calcium and displaces calcium in the bones, leaving them weakened and prone to fracture. This explains why I went from maximum bone density to extreme osteoporosis. Mercury is a neurotoxin that can affect the GI tract, the kidneys, and the nervous system; it can also interrupt the electrical circuits of the sinus node that control heart beats. This explains my arrhythmia.[4] Then there is arsenic, exposure to which produces serious effects on the neurologic, respiratory, hematologic, and cardiovascular systems, and which acts as a carcinogen in multiple organ systems.[5]

Time for Action

Now that I had the most probable cause of my symptoms, I immediately made plans to have my implants removed. I had the explant surgery on May 17, 2019, and although not all of the issues have resolved, I have steadily improved. I started researching ways to get the silicone and heavy metals out of my body. So far, there doesn't seem to be any way to get the silicone out because it gets imbedded in the organs, including the brain, and removal of vital organs is hardly a possibility.

There is, however, something I can do about the residual heavy metals, with the help of the organs of detoxification—the liver, kidneys, colon, lungs, and skin. I knew that being on the diet I was already on is the best way to support all of these organs, especially the liver, kidneys, and colon. Moreover, it seems logical to assume that exercising vigorously, thus inducing heavy breathing, is the best way to support the lungs, and that sweating is the best way to take advantage of the skin's detoxing abilities (a process that is greatly increased in efficiency by the use of a sauna).

Based on her research on using nutrition to reverse autoimmune diseases including lupus, Brooke Goldner, MD advised me to follow the protocol that she had studied.[6] She agreed that my diet was good but suggested that it could be more effective if I increased my intake of leafy greens by incorporating green smoothies. My thrice-daily green smoothies now contain kale, Swiss chard, cilantro, and any one of the many varieties of cabbage, plus ginger, flaxseeds, chia seeds, and garlic. One carafe-ful makes up about a third of each meal and ensures a near-continuous availability of the powerful nutrients that I need to regain my health.

I Was Not Alone

Along with my personal revelation, I discovered that there were thousands upon thousands of women who were suffering from similar symptoms from their breast implants, whether from post-mastectomy reconstruction or cosmetic breast enlargement. There are now several online forums such as the Facebook group Fierce, Flat, Forward, which consists of women who previously had mastectomies due to breast cancer, who have removed their implants and refused further reconstruction. We are proudly flat.

I kept my eyes open for any further research to get more answers since I knew those fifteen specialists I'd seen probably still believed that silicone implants were safe. After all, the FDA had decreed that they were made of medical-grade silicone, inert, tested, and approved for use in the human body. Most doctors still have not gotten the word on the reality.

Since then, I have found two published medical-journal articles on the topic.

Guilty as Charged

September 2020
Silicone Breast Implants—Historical Medical Error

Abstract

Silicone is a foreign material to our body and therefore has been found to stimulate the immune system. Silicone breast implants (SBIs), made of silicone polymer, have been used for aesthetic and medical purposes since the 1960s, and were found to trigger acute/chronic inflammation, eventually leading to the formation of fibrotic capsules on the surface of the implant. Silicone implants have been found to be associated with the development of severe and sometimes unexplained clinical manifestations such as: chronic fatigue, sleep and memory problems, widespread pain, dry mouth and eyes, depression, arthralgia, myalgia, palpitations, tinnitus and hearing loss, skin rash, hair loss, vision problems, hyperhidrosis, allergic reactions, etc. Furthermore, SBIs have been found to be associated with the development of rheumatologic/autoimmune diseases and the development of rare lymphoma. The FDA has expressed concern over the years about the implications of SBIs and requested that the companies involved provide data of any concern regarding the implants. However, the companies continued to sell the implants without reporting data, as agreed. In October 2019, the FDA recommended boxed warnings describing the dangers facing women applying for SBIs such as lymphoma. Importantly, our lab recently found the presence of autoantibodies against the autonomic nervous system in the blood of women with SBIs, which might explain some of the patients' severe symptoms. Owing to the numerous data that had been accumulated (since 1960s) indicating a direct link between silicone, autoimmune diseases and cancer, we believe that the use of SBIs has been a historical medical error.

And more evidence follows two years later:

January 2022
Breast Implant Illness: Scientific Evidence of Its Existence

Abstract

More than one million breast augmentation procedures using silicone breast implants (SBI) have been performed worldwide. Adverse events of SBI include local complications such as pain, swelling, redness, infections, capsular contracture, implant rupture, and gel-bleed. Furthermore, patients experience systemic symptoms such as chronic fatigue, arthralgias, myalgias, pyrexia, sicca, and cognitive dysfunction. These symptoms received different names such as autoimmune/autoinflammatory syndrome induced by adjuvants (ASIA) due to silicone incompatibility syndrome and breast implant illness (BII). Because of chronic immune activation, BII/ASIA, allergies, autoimmune diseases, immune deficiencies, and finally lymphomas may develop in SBI patients.

Alternatives after Mastectomy

Because the immune system immediately recognizes anything that qualifies as a foreign body, the attack begins on day one as acute inflammation, which continues, becoming chronic, until that foreign body is removed. Obviously, silicone breast implants are impervious to attacks by the immune system and the "war" continues as long as those implants remain in the body. There are drugs that can disable your immune system but which, as a consequence, leave you vulnerable to bacteria, viruses, fungi, and cancer cells.

Breast cancer patients who have undergone mastectomies, who will not consider going flat but are aware of the dangers of silicone implants, can choose the alternative of having their own body tissues used to surgically replicate breast mounds. As mentioned earlier, either stomach fat or tissue from the latissimus muscle from the back is transferred to the chest area and formed into the new breasts. Neither of these procedures interested me in the least as I did not want more surgery. I now believe that following mastectomy to treat breast cancer, there is no need for "reconstruction," that the body is still perfect even if somewhat amended. I no longer have the "killer breasts" that tried twice to kill me, although the remaining silicone may still succeed. I not-so-jokingly tell the fifteen specialists of old to put on my gravestone, "I told you so!"

My philosophy now is encompassed by this line from Dr. Seuss: "When something bad happens to you, you have three choices. You can either let it define you, let it destroy you, or let it strengthen you."

I'm a warrior who now wears her battle scars proudly.

CHAPTER NINETEEN

THE IRONMAN: KONA, HAWAII

The tiny village of Kona on the Big Island of Hawaii gets transformed every October as the Ironman competitors start arriving. The air is absolutely electric with the tension among the triathletes, so many of whom are dead serious. The pier at Alii Drive connects the start and finish of the swim leg and the start of the 112-mile bike leg. From Kona to Hawi, 56 desolate, deserted, hot, black, lava-covered miles lie in wait for poor, unsuspecting cyclists. After the turnaround at Hawi, another 56 miles, desolate, deserted, and now windy, await. The last few miles of the bike leg give competitors a short but welcome relief as they roll downhill to Keahou Beach Hotel. That's where the bikes get dropped off for the immediate switch to running shoes, with the clock still running. The marathon run starts at Keahou Beach Hotel and routes competitors back to the pier at the end of Alii Drive.

Once out of the Kona village, runners, by now exhausted, have to traverse the same desolation for the 10 miles to the marathon turnaround, past the airport. There is nothing but deadly heat and boredom. One tedious mile after another seems to just suck the energy, bodily fluids, and determination right out of the most committed of competitors. For the entire final 6 miles in between Keahou Beach Hotel and Alii Drive, there are parked cars and throngs of cheering spectators along the roads with homemade, locally appropriate expressions of their support and whatever kind of aid is necessary and compliant with the rules. At the other end of Alii Drive, 26.2 miles later, is the finale, the finish line for the Ironman triathlon.

These are the images that were going through my head all week long just before my sixth Ironman. I felt strong enough to continue hard training, but I knew that I had to "taper," as triathletes say—to ease off on the hardest miles of training so that my body could recover its energy and strength. A very common mistake triathletes make is to go into a race not completely recovered from their last hard training session.

Yet I found it difficult to taper when I had so much energy. I just couldn't sit still. We triathletes always say, "I'll start my taper now." Then we end up going for "just a short swim to loosen up the shoulders," "just a short bike ride to loosen up the legs," or "just a short run to get rid of some excess energy." Of course, once we start, it's like taking "just one potato chip." It can't be done!

Thou Shalt Know the Course

There are competitors swimming the evening before a triathlon; there are also those who arrive so late that they have no choice but to check things out—the swim, bike, and run courses—at practically the last minute. Either way, one of the cardinal rules of racing is: know the course.

This is especially true of the Kona Ironman, particularly as there are competitors arriving from all over the world, many of whom have never even been to America, much less Kona, Hawaii. This obviously presents quite a problem when the course covers so many miles, to say nothing of the frequently extreme conditions. One year, the winds were so strong that they literally blew cyclists off their bikes. Likewise, the ocean can be so rough that swimmers get too seasick to continue, as their vomiting sucks the strength right out of their bodies. And if you're a runner, you know what 114-degree-Fahrenheit weather can do to you.

Needless to say, newly arrived competitors are anxious about the course. You cannot even check out the course in the cool of the evening without grave risk since there aren't any streetlights along Alii Drive. The date of the Ironman is selected on the basis of the lunar calendar, and competitors have until midnight to finish. The light of a full moon is all there is to guide many on their quest for the finish line.

Feelings of nervousness and anxiety were constantly welling up within me. Despite continuously reminding myself that I had done an Ironman several times before and could therefore do it again, I still felt extremely apprehensive. I almost envied the first-timers: after all, they did not yet know how bad it could get out there. I also knew that for each of my five previous Ironman events, given all the things that could have gone wrong, the odds had been in my favor; one of these days, those odds were going to catch up with me.

Some of my fears centered on possible mechanical problems with the bike. I rode racing wheels with twelve spokes in front and eighteen on the rear. (The usual number of spokes is thirty-six.) This concession to aerodynamics and light weight did not inspire confidence in me or anyone who looked at my wheels, usually with great amazement. "Those wheels don't look like they could hold you up," or, "You've got more guts than I do, lady," the skeptics would say. I had been assured, however, that they were as strong as—if not stronger than—conventional, thirty-six–spoked wheels. And so far, they'd served me well. Five Ironman triathlons without a mishap or even getting out of true (alignment)!

There was an incident in one of the races when I thought I had a problem. I was coming down the home stretch of the bicycle leg, concentrating only on keeping up my speed. All of a sudden, there was a *tick-tick-tick* with each revolution of my front wheel. I was near panic. Expecting the wheel to collapse at any moment, I put on my brakes, trying to slow down so that when I fell, I wouldn't hit the pavement so hard. Then I thought of stopping to try to fix the problem. All the insecurities I'd ever had about my limited prowess as a mechanic came surging at me. I took the cowardly way out and kept pedaling. The ticking continued unabated but nothing else was happening. With my heart in my throat, I decided to get as close to the bike finish line as possible so as to cut down the distance I would have to carry my bike to the bike transition point. (Triathlon rules say only that you and your bike have to finish; you don't have to be on it. You could carry it!)

By this time, my legs were rubbery and shaking as the panic-induced adrenaline was wearing off. I was, to say the least, a nervous wreck. But still, nothing was happening. The wheels were still turning, and I was still upright on the bike. Finally, the finish line was in sight. I pushed myself for an extra surge of speed, crossed the finish line, dropped the bike, and took off running. It was only on completion of the run that I found out what had happened. The sensor of my speedometer had loosened its attachment to the spoke and had been dangling uselessly, hitting the brake with every revolution of the wheel. You can bet that I now frequently check for loose screws on the connector for that errant sensor!

Then there are all the things that can go wrong during the marathon leg. Every time I consider just those 26.2 miles alone, forgetting for a moment the 2.4 miles of swimming and 112 miles of cycling, I still shake my head in disbelief. The thought that logically, it can't be done keeps cropping up, especially when I recall some of my 100-mile training rides and the 112-mile Around-Oahu Bike Race, at the end of which I could barely limp into the finish area.

What racing has taught me is that we do what we have to do. When I program my mind for the task ahead, this will *generally* (and I stress this word) keep my body going until the end—whenever that end comes. This is how I cope with differing external and internal conditions. What I see is what I get, and I just get on with it. This plan is not always foolproof, as I am reminded periodically when I see a burned-out competitor staggering, zombie-like, in directions not always leading directly to the finish line.

What's even more heart-rending is to see a fallen athlete like the iconic Julie Moss whom I mentioned in an earlier chapter, who, then in first place, collapsed and, with an extreme will and the encouragement of the cheering crowd, literally crawled to the finish line. It brings tears to my eyes as I wonder how our minds can push our bodies to and even beyond their physical limits. What a demonstration of the power of the mind—of its ability to set goals, to visualize the attainment of said goals, and to perform what must be self-hypnosis! I still oftentimes marvel at the genius of our species. We're all pretty incredible when you stop to think about it.

The Sleep of the Exhausted

One thing that many competitors have noticed is that although the pre-race anxiety may be pretty devastating, we can usually sleep very well. No matter how nervous I am about an ultra-distance event, I've at least gotten a decent night's sleep the night before. Sometimes, I can hardly hold my eyelids open past 9 p.m. The only thing is that when I'm really nervous, I tend to wake up early. Since most races start at very early hours, however, this works out well.

Of course, with the heavy training required to compete, you tend to sleep very soundly, and it's important to get your seven to nine hours of sleep. In addition to a challenging exercise load and an extremely healthy diet, I believe that all bodily systems work better with the important recovery and resilience gained from enough high-quality sleep.

As it turns out, all the insecurities that flooded my mind during the week preceding the Kona Ironman served a very useful purpose: they kept me from getting overconfident. You should never take an event like an Ironman lightly, no matter how many times you've done it. Even if your conditioning is as good as or better than in past events, there are always different conditions on the course. While it's true that the experience you've gained helps, no two events are ever identical, nor are you ever overprepared for all of the risky situations that could come up.

Life Is Not Always Fair

Two weeks before the 1987 Kona Ironman, a competitor was hit by a concrete truck and killed. I knew the incredible Pat Griskus, having ridden alongside him in the 1986 Ironman when we were both trying to buoy each other's resolve to keep going at the 80-mile mark of the bike leg. Pat had lost a leg in a motorcycle accident some years prior. He had gotten an artificial leg, put running shoes on, and set out to compete in the Ironman. The thought that if Pat could make it, so must I had been my inspiration for the race. It was beyond tragic that he did not make it after all that he'd been through.

In the 1986 event, I had been riding out in the middle of the lava fields at temperatures over 100 degrees Fahrenheit and was experiencing a terrible low. I wanted to get off my bike in the worst way and go stretch out on the lava. Reminding myself that rough, hot lava was no place to lie down, I negotiated with myself to try to keep going until I reached the next aid station. Then, I reasoned, I could lie down where there would be medical aid if I needed it. But the lava kept enticing me. I had to keep telling myself that it was *not* a big, soft, fluffy, cushy chocolate marshmallow but hard, searing-hot, black molten rock. I must have been hallucinating!

Checking my mileage, I calculated that the next aid station was only a couple of miles away. *Surely*, I thought, *if Pat can keep going, then so can I.* I ought to be able to make it to that point, and *then* I could lie down. I started to wonder why I was putting myself through this agony. It had never happened before. Maybe people were right—three to four Ironman triathlons in a year are too much for any body. Then I recalled that I had not eaten any real food since the start of the race, relying instead on liquid supplements that were supposed to provide calories, electrolytes, and fluids.

When I finally made it to the next aid station, I gobbled up everything in sight: bananas, an orange, some cookies, and I can't remember what else. Within a few minutes, I could feel the energy coursing through my body. I now felt as if I could make it to the next aid station before lying down. When I reached that aid station as well, I thought that I would be able to at least finish the bike leg. When I finally got to the end of the bike leg, I thought that I could run just a couple of miles to make it a "complete" training day; I'd surely lie down then.

After a few miles, I realized that I was feeling strong enough to take on the marathon. I could not believe it myself! I'd gone from one extreme to the other—from first wanting desperately to lie down on a bed of hot lava to completing the marathon and crossing the finish line of the whole race, feeling so fantastic that I babbled on euphorically for several hours after.

That is the memory I have of the last Ironman Pat and I both took part in, during which we both questioned our sanity for even being out there, doing these painful things to our bodies. As I stared in disbelief at the newspaper article announcing his death, the shock hit hard. It was not the first time something like this had happened, I realized, and it could happen to any one of us at any time. After all, I had come close, getting hit by a truck in 1984 and again in 1998.

Are we crazy for exposing ourselves to such high risk? Are we playing Russian roulette with our lives? Well, what are the odds? If there are 1,500 competitors and one gets killed, is this a reason for the rest to back out of the competition? Is not daily living risky to one degree or another? Where do we put ourselves on the risk continuum? I suppose one is exposed to the least amount of risk when confined to one's own bedroom; even the kitchen and the bathroom are where many accidents occur. Does it make any sense to say that we should therefore spend our whole lives in our bedrooms? Obviously not. Then there's the other extreme, at which we are placing ourselves in constant danger. I guess the answer lies somewhere in between. We each have to determine how much risk we are willing to take in our lives. Without risk, there can be no gain; we have to put ourselves on the start line first. The number-one rule is: just show up.

It's a fact of life that people are more frequently sorry for what they did *not* do—a risk they did *not* take—than they are for anything they ever did. I am not an exception. So while I'm not saying that everybody should get out there and ride bicycles on busy highways or do an Ironman, I am glad that I've taken the particular risks that I have in life.

Being diagnosed with breast cancer has made me more of a risk-taker. For one, I've often felt that I had nothing to lose—I was going to die anyway. Of course, we will all die eventually; the only question is when and how. In my case, my diagnosis gave me a probable "how" but not a "when." So my thinking became: *if I'm going to go, I'm going to have done something worthwhile first.*

Now, Forty Years Out

Now, as I come up on over forty years since my diagnosis, my mind conjures up two starkly contrasting images. One is of me at the age of a hundred, having experienced no recurrence of cancer and reversed the horrible breast-implant illness. I imagine I would feel sad that I had wasted so much time worrying, so much time on all the doctor's visits and tests, that I had let the specter of cancer shadow the things I'd done.

Then my mind goes to the immediate future. Maybe tomorrow will be the day when I feel that something's wrong and go get tested, then the hospital calls to say that I need to see my doctor, that they can't tell me the results over the phone. If this happens, I would feel the despair of losing the good feelings of invulnerability that have been slowly reforming in my mind as I got further away from the day of that deadly diagnosis. So which is it to be? This says a lot for living in the present moment (what I call "awarenessing"), doesn't it? We must make each day count because that really is all we have.

A lot of these thoughts came up whenever I was in the midst of a long race. There were times when the present moment was extremely uncomfortable and I wondered why I was putting myself through it. People ask the same questions when they are in any stage of life where there is discomfort. The Ironman is a symbolic representation of life, a microcosm of a lifetime. There are highs and lows in between the start and finish of an event, but there's nothing like getting the reward at the end. What that reward looks like is different for each one of us.

For me, each time when I have crossed a finish line, I have felt a mixture of joy and excitement that immediately canceled out all the discomfort I'd felt just moments before. I would then walk around to see those who came in before me and to share their joy. Next, I would get to greet those just coming in and celebrate with them as they crossed the finish line. I am reminded of the sheer value of racing, in an Ironman triathlon or otherwise, every time I finish a race and, after a short recovery period, am ready to jump in again, eagerly declaring, "Just wait 'til next time!" And every "next time" has just gotten better and better. I wish it never has to end.

Chapter Twenty

What's the Prognosis? Why Cancer Isn't Curable

Cancer is a very scary disease. Even after the world has experienced the likes of AIDS and COVID-19, it is still the disease that people fear the most. It is also about to overtake heart disease as the number-one cause of death in the US. A mention of cancer usually conjures up an image of a patient who will be ravaged by chemotherapy and radiation, then die despite the treatment.

Newspapers and magazines regularly report on "breakthroughs" in cancer treatments and claims of "longer" survival times. In reality, it is just that with better screening and diagnostic techniques, patients now find out about their cancer earlier, and so their survival times are artificially lengthened even though the natural course of the disease in most cases is still unfortunately the same. It's often at least eight to ten years before cancer is clinically detectable by the usual methods, and by that time, the cancerous tumor that started from a single cell has had time to grow.

It's the nature of cancer to create its own blood supply via angiogenesis, thereby shedding cancer cells that are carried throughout the body. It's almost impossible to detect the new colonies until they, too, are large enough to be picked up by blood tests, x-rays, scans such as MRIs, and the likes. For chemotherapy and radiation to kill all of the cancer cells, the doses have to be so high that they nearly kill the patient. These treatments can cause irreversible damage to the patient's heart, lungs, and most importantly, immune system, which, after all, is what keeps them alive. Without our immune systems, we are prey to every little bug that comes along.

What's confusing to a lot of people is how cancer kills. Right after my diagnosis, the macho guys in the office where I worked said, "Well, come on, it's just a breast." They had no idea that it's not the primary (first) tumor

186

discovered that is fatal, especially in the case of breast, colon, prostate, and some skin cancers. It's the metastasis (spread) of the cancer cells, which break off and set up housekeeping in the liver, bones, lungs, and brain. It's exactly like letting *all* of the horses out of the barn. Tracking down these rogue cells is extremely difficult, and shooting them down with chemicals and radiation is not only difficult but also exceedingly hazardous to normal cells. That's why chemotherapy and radiation treatments cause nausea, vomiting, and hair loss. The normal cells most vulnerable to these weapons are the fastest-growing cells, those in the lining of the gastrointestinal system and in hair. If the treatment is not powerful enough to cause the side effects, it's not likely to stop any cancer cells either.

Because oncologists (cancer specialists) are seeing so little change in the life expectancies of patients with the most common cancers, many are finally starting to emphasize prevention. Based on epidemiological population studies, it is very clear that different countries have unique frequencies of the different kinds of cancer. When many of these frequencies are correlated with dietary habits, a telling pattern emerges.

Indeed, based on the evidence, many researchers are now convinced that breast, prostate, and colon cancers are related to diet. There is an almost-perfect correlation between rate of death from breast cancer and percentage of dietary fat (the primary source of which is animal foods), according to findings by researcher Ken Carroll way back in 1975.[1]

Then, in 1977, A. Lowenthals published a study showing that the incidences of breast and colon cancers were on the rise together in fifty-six countries of the world.[2] Further, when you look at the similarity in the rising and falling of the cancer rates and dietary fat intake, it is striking that nearly all of the variance is explained. In other words, there isn't room left for other variables, including genetics and environmental factors such as stress.

But if genetics doesn't play a role, what about the breast cancer genes, BRCA1 and BRCA2? We now know a lot more about epigenetics and the ability of lifestyle, in particular diet, to turn genes on and off. The analogy is that the genes load the gun and the lifestyle pulls the trigger. When it's so obvious to me that animal products can turn on the cancer genes, I am all the sadder when I read about women undergoing prophylactic mastectomies when they find out they have BRCA1 and BRCA2. In my own case, I was advised to opt for a prophylactic mastectomy on my left breast since I was at a "very high risk of cancer" in that breast; I ended up agreeing to what I now feel was unnecessary surgery. I think the evidence is clear that a diet totally devoid of animal-based foods and of oils makes the "cancerous trigger" far more unlikely to be pulled.

The same analogy applies to dementia and Alzheimer's disease. If you have the APOE gene, that's the loaded gun, whereas research is showing that it's lifestyle, primarily poor diet and lack of exercise, that pulls the trigger. On the other hand, a low-fat, whole-food, plant-based diet and regular exercise help prevent the trigger from being pulled altogether. If you've made it this far in this book, you know that these two things also help protect you against heart disease, stroke, diabetes, high blood pressure, obesity, erectile dysfunction, kidney failure, and much more.

By the way, when I tell people who have type 2 diabetes that they can reverse it by changing to a vegan, whole-food, plant-based diet, they don't believe me. Often, their response is, "Diabetes runs in my family," to which I say, "Oh no, it's the *diet* that runs in your family."

Check out the current research in this area to see how medical doctors who specialize in lifestyle medicine are using diet to reverse so many of the most common degenerative diseases.

Nature's Experiment

While we can't carry out the live human experiments that we would need to prove our theory, we can take advantage of the natural experiment that has been provided to us—if only we are smart enough to look at the data. The few countries whose populations eat more fat than we do in the US—the Netherlands, Denmark, and New Zealand, for example—also have higher rates of death from breast cancer.

As early as 1963, Ernst Wynder, MD, founder and president of the American Health Foundation, already noted the fact that Japanese women with breast cancer living in Japan survived much longer than did American breast cancer patients. You can dismiss the role of genetics here because Americans of Japanese ancestry who suffered from breast cancer died at the same rate as did other American patients due to their following the SAD diet.[3]

There are other cancer types with dismal survival rates. Lung cancer, for example, has a five-year survival rate of less than 10 percent, meaning that fewer than one out of ten people are alive five years after their diagnosis. The Surgeon General's Report in 1979 indicated that little significant progress in the diagnosis or treatment of lung cancer had been made in the previous fifteen years.[4] Little has changed since then, and the mortality rate of lung cancer in women surpassed that of breast cancer in 1987, clearly reflecting the increased number of women who smoked.

When I did the Japan Ironman in 1986, I found it disturbing that after I crossed the finish line along with many of the male competitors, the first thing they did was light up cigarettes. In fact, when reporters came to interview me, the smoke was so thick that I was fanning some away from my face. I asked if we could move away from the smoke. Surprised that this bothered me at all, they nevertheless agreed. From this incident, I thought for sure that lung cancer rates in Japan would be high but then found out that the disease was rare there. Dr. McDougall explained to me that Japanese people's healthier diet gave them some protection from carcinogens. Of course, this was back in the 1980s, when their diet was still based mostly on rice. Sadly, this has changed, and I have been told that Japan now even has to deal with "chubby children."

If we could rule out two of the most preventable causes of cancer, an animal-based diet and smoking, we would eliminate most of the cancers (not just lung cancer) in the US and in the West. (The remaining types of cancer, the relatively rare ones, are yielding to new advances in cancer therapies.) Wouldn't it be great if we had a magic wand with which we could just wave animal foods and cigarettes out of people's lives?

Why There May Never Be a Cure for Cancer

More than fifty years since former president Richard Nixon declared a war on cancer and the search for its cure, there still is no chemotherapy, radiation therapy, hormone blocker, or surgery that can guarantee no recurrence and a permanent cancer-free state. Cancer is much like the viruses that cause pandemics, ever mutating and ever evading the vaccines that we keep developing to target specific new strains. Viruses are wily and develop ways to hide behind our immune systems, waiting to attack again. This is true of cancer cells, which are no less wily and also develop immunity to all the defenses we throw at them.

There are neoadjuvant therapies, such as biologics, that are implemented before adjuvant therapies (chemotherapy, radiation, and hormone therapy) with the purpose of shrinking tumors to make them more operable, reducing the need for mastectomies, and killing cancer cells that have spread. Again, all of these treatments only increase the likelihood of and do not guarantee survival. Billions of dollars will continue to be thrown at Big Pharma for research and development of new therapies. But only when that money is invested in tackling the *root* causes of most cancers, primarily an animal-based diet and smoking, will real progress be made in Nixon's war against cancer and the futile search for a cure be rendered obsolete!

Given that this scenario is impossible in the near future, there is an alternative that works: make athletes out of all meat-eaters and smokers! Once an individual starts an athletic training program, they often find it easier to take better care of themselves. They will quit smoking and start eating a healthier diet, losing unwanted weight, feeling and looking better, and perhaps even competing in races. Any or all of these outcomes positively reinforce their training program. They usually will no longer have any desire to do anything that is counterproductive to being a winner.

This means that the person wins, the body wins, society wins, the animals win, and the environment wins—nobody loses! There is no greater "high" than that of doing well in the race for life. And doing well here doesn't necessarily mean placing first. For beginners, it means just finishing the race. For the more advanced, it means setting a personal record—finishing in a shorter time than ever before. I've seen people jump up and down, scream, and generally go wild when they've set a new PR. It's that exciting for them. Then, placing first can illicit joy, excitement, and pride that last for years. Plus, such an achievement is usually made more tangible by a cool trophy or plaque.

Now, this is not to say that success comes easy. There is discomfort, sometimes even pain. There were times during Ironman competitions when I felt extreme pain—pain so intense that I wondered what the point of it all was.

What I have learned from all of the races, however, is that when I cross a finish line, all of a sudden, the pain gets washed away by euphoric joy. I never realized how intense that feeling could be until I saw a photograph of me at the finish line of my first Ironman. I was amazed at the expression on my face. I had never seen a look so ecstatic—a look that has been reproduced in every finish-line photo ever since.

Scientists have postulated that this euphoria is caused by endorphins, chemicals the body makes that are similar to opiates and that make us feel good at such times. Regardless, whether it's the endorphins or the purely intellectual joy of having accomplished a major goal is irrelevant. What *is* relevant is that what is going on here psychologically has implications for disease survival.

Why Some Make It and Some Don't

One of the great mysteries of cancer (and other diseases as well) is why some people survive when they were not expected to and some die when they were expected to survive. If you remember, in my case, the doctors at first could not tell me whether I had three months, three years, or three decades to live. Even the multiple "second" opinions I got were not any more illuminating.

In their book *Getting Well Again*, Stephanie and O. Carl Simonton promote the theory that it boils down to whether or not a patient has a strong enough determination to fight their disease.[5] What's more is that this will to survive seems to be bolstered by visualizations of the body's immune system actively engaging the disease in combat. As I trained over hundreds of hours, rhythmically paddling, pedaling, and plodding, I was probably in a state of intense focus; I was in the zone—as they say—or a self-hypnotic trance. I was giving myself suggestions about how I was getting stronger, healthier, and more efficient at helping my white blood cells kill cancer cells.

Visualization is a relatively passive process. You're supposed to sit or lie quietly and picture strong, powerful white blood cells searching for and destroying confused, weak cancer cells. While working at this, I found myself gritting my teeth, trying to make the visualization more "real." I tried, through closed eyes, to "see" my white blood cells gobbling up vagrant cancer cells. All I really saw was a velvety purple, with flashes here and there, as my squinting put pressure on my optic nerve.

It is a different matter on the playing field, however, where visualization becomes an active process. What an understatement to call doing an Ironman "active"! Here I am, spending an entire day and part of a night swimming, biking, and running at race pace, feeling exhilarated, healthy, and in total control of my universe. These feelings for me are very real. No visualization is required. I'm on the move, on the offense, and in complete control of my life, being as far from passive as one can get.

As the feelings of fatigue start to creep up on me, I'm still battling on, except that now, the "enemy" is real. My body is obeying all of my commands to race for time—to win the race and to win in life. My body is functioning at its best because I provide it with the right fuel. That's part of the fun too: you burn up around 10,000 calories doing an Ironman. I'm experiencing the full range of human emotions, getting a glimpse of a microcosm of a lifetime, and gaining a perspective of who I am and what I want out of life. That, I suppose, could be called "active" visualization.

Taking Control

All of this has to be good for the immune system in the long run. In the short run, intense physical activity may temporarily depress the white blood cell count. For me, doing the Ironman was my way of taking control of my disease. Instead of doing nothing or grasping at chemotherapy, radiation, and other possible cures, I was being as active as I possibly could. This is only my hypothesis, but I think that the perceived loss of control that accompanies a diagnosis of cancer is one of the deadliest aspects of this disease. The only way I could counter that feeling and wrest control again was by aiming for the Ironman.

Counseling cancer patients over the years, I've observed that about 20 percent of people who are seriously ill would give up and die if given the opportunity. About 60 percent are willing to live provided that the doctors do the work and the treatment is not too uncomfortable. The final 20 percent say: "I'll do anything to get well. Just tell me what to do!"

This book, with the program herein, was written for people in the last category. It was also written for those who have not yet been diagnosed with a serious illness but, if they had, would have fallen into the last 20 percent. And in any case, people who follow this program will probably be successful in avoiding the three major yet preventable killers of Americans—cancer, heart disease, and stroke. I hope you are one of them.

The discoveries I have made along my multi-decade journey to Ironman triathlons have been exciting and revolutionary. At first, the medical community was totally against the idea that diet, exercise, and mental fortitude could possibly make a difference in a cancer patient's chances of survival. Little by little, I was feeling my way. As I increased my exercise, I found my ability to take control increasing as well. This also served as my psychological support. At the same time, I started to see external validation in the press—glimmerings of increasing awareness of the role of diet and exercise in the treatment of cancer.

A year into this program, I got a letter from two Ohio State University researchers with a request to fill out a questionnaire about my exercise. They were onto the same thing I was. Another year went by, then I got a phone call from a national running magazine reporter in New York City (remember, I'm in Hawaii) who'd heard about my unusual approach to dealing with cancer. The interview we ended up doing culminated in a very nice story on me, which was to be followed by articles in *Newsday, USA Today, Honolulu Star-Bulletin, The Honolulu Advertiser*, and international publications such as the *New Zealand Herald*, Japan's *Asahi Shimbun*, Australia's running magazine *The Fun Runner*, in addition to newspaper blurbs all over the US and in Russia, Thailand, and Nepal. *Runner's World* magazine also presented me with their Golden Shoe Award.

The positive research results keep coming out. More recently, different published studies have suggested that regular physical activity is associated with a lower risk for several types of cancer, including breast, prostate, colon, endometrium, and possibly pancreatic cancers.[6] Additionally, active women have been shown to have about half the rates of lymphoma, leukemia, myeloma, Hodgkin's disease, and cancer of the thyroid compared to their sedentary counterparts. The same is true for other, less common types of cancer.[7]

While these results say a lot about what can be done before one ever gets a diagnosis, what is clear to me is that whatever prevents cancer logically will help control and halt the spread of cancer once it's established in the body. Some oncologists now believe that factors that initiate cancer also promote it, and diet is definitely one such factor.

In sum, does my approach work? A study by C. Barber Mueller, MD way back in 1978 showed that 88 percent of breast cancer patients who nonetheless died of other causes still had breast cancer cells in their bodies, based on data collected over nineteen years by the Syracuse, NY, Upstate Medical Center Cancer Registry on 3,558 women.[8] Since cancer cells can remain viable in vitro (in the laboratory) for up to fifty years, it's too soon to tell if my approach is working. Besides, an "experiment" with a sample of one is totally inadequate and considered just an anecdote. We need more controlled studies to show that diet can make a difference in disease survival rates, corroborating the experimental findings we already have.[9] What I hope my story can do, in the meantime, is point the way for others.

If you really want to live the "good" life, with "good" food and "good" exercise, and get yourself as fit as you can (or what I call "super-fit"), use this three-pronged approach—consisting of a whole-food, plant-based, no-oil diet, effective exercise, and active visualization—and give it all you've got! It's a race worth winning!

NOTES

Introduction

1. Jin-Soo Kim, Rebekah L. Wilson, Dennis R. Taaffe, Daniel A. Galvão, Elin Gray, and Robert U. Newton, "Myokine Expression and Tumor-Suppressive Effect of Serum after 12 wk of Exercise in Prostate Cancer Patients on ADT," *Medicine and Science in Sports and Exercise* 54, no. 2 (Febuary 1, 2022): 197–205, https://pubmed.ncbi.nlm.nih.gov/34559721/.

Chapter One

1. Francis Collins, "Americans Are Still Eating Too Much Added Sugar, Fat," *NIH Director's Blog*, October 1, 2019, https://directorsblog.nih.gov/2019/10/01/americans-are-still-eating-too-much-added-sugar-fat/.
2. Rin Ogiya et al., "Breast Cancer Survival among Japanese Individuals and US Residents of Japanese and Other Origins: A Comparative Registry-Based Study," *Breast Cancer Research and Treatment* 184, no. 2 (August 20, 2020), doi:10.1007/s10549-020-05869-y.
3. David Grotto and Elisa Zied, "The Standard American Diet and Its Relationship to the Health Status of Americans," *Nutrition in Clinical Practice* 25, no. 6 (2010): 603–12, doi:10.1177/0884533610386234.

Chapter Three

1. Karl Sabbagh, "The Psychopathology of Fringe Medicine," *The Skeptical Inquirer* 10, no. 2 (Winter 1985), https://skepticalinquirer.org/1986/01/the-psychopathology-of-fringe-medicine/.
2. Walter C. Willett et al., "Dietary Fat and Fiber in Relation to Risk of Breast Cancer: An 8-Year Follow-Up," *JAMA* 268, no. 15 (October 21, 1992): 2037–44, doi:10.1001/jama.1992.03490150089030.
3. Victor W. Zhong et al., "Associations of Dietary Cholesterol or Egg Consumption with Incident Cardiovascular Disease and Mortality," *JAMA* 321, no. 11 (March 19, 2019): 1081–95, doi:10.1001/jama.2019.1572.

4.   Rikki A. Cannioto et al., "Physical Activity Before, During, and after Chemotherapy for High-Risk Breast Cancer: Relationships with Survival," *Journal of the National Cancer Institute* 113, no. 1 (January 4, 2021): 54–63, doi:10.1093/jnci/djaa046.

5.   Zhilei Shan et al., "Healthy Eating Patterns and Risk of Total and Cause-Specific Mortality," *JAMA Internal Medicine* 183, no. 2 (January 9, 2023): 142–53, doi:10.1001/jamainternmed.2022.6117.

6.   Hyunju Kim et al., "Plant-Based Diets, Pescatarian Diets and COVID-19 Severity: A Population-Based Case-Control Study in Six Countries," *BMJ Nutrition, Prevention and Health* (June 7, 2021), doi: 10.1136/bmjnph-2021-000272.

Chapter Five

1.   Denis P. Burkitt, "Colonic-Rectal Cancer: Fiber and Other Dietary Factors," *The American Journal of Clinical Nutrition* 31, no. 10 (October 1978): S58–64, doi:10.1093/ajcn/31.10.S58.

2.   Shaneerra Raajlynn Kaur Sidhu, Chin Wei Kok, Thubasni Kunasegaran, and Amutha Ramadas, "Effect of Plant-Based Diets on Gut Microbiota: A Systematic Review of Interventional Studies," *Nutrients* 15, no. 6 (March 1, 2023): 1510, doi:10.3390/nu15061510.

3.   Andrea Grillo, Lucia Salvi, Paolo Coruzzi, Paolo Salvi, and Gianfranco Parati, "Sodium Intake and Hypertension," *Nutrients* 11, no. 9 (September 2019): 1970, doi:10.3390/nu11091970.

4.   T Colin Campbell, "A Study on Diet, Nutrition, and Disease in the People's Republic of China: Part I," *Boletin de la Asociacion Medica de Puerto Rico* 82, no. 3 (1990): 132–4, https://pubmed.ncbi.nlm.nih.gov/2322353/.

5.   Kelly A. Barrett et al., "Fish-Associated Foodborne Disease Outbreaks: United States, 1998–2015," *Foodborne Pathogens and Disease* 14, no. 9 (2017): 537–43, doi:10.1089/fpd.2017.2286.

6.   Marjo H. Eskelinen and Miia Kivipelto, "Caffeine as a Protective Factor in Dementia and Alzheimer's Disease," *Journal of Alzheimer's Disease* 20, suppl. 1 (2010): S167–74, doi:10.3233/JAD-2010-1404.

7.   Ibid.

8.   Lori Uildriks, "Microplastics in Humans: After Blood, Scientists Find Traces in the Lungs," *Medical News Today*, April 12, 2022, https://www.medicalnewstoday.com/articles/microplastics-in-humans-after-blood-scientists-find-traces-in-the-lungs.

9.   United Nations, "Rearing Cattle Produces More Greenhouse Gases than Driving Cars, UN Report Warns," *UN News*, November 29, 2006, https://news.un.org/en/story/2006/11/201222-rearing-cattle-produces-more-greenhouse-gases-driving-cars-un-report-warns.

Chapter Six

1. David McNamee, "Running for Exercise 'Slows the Aging Process,'" *Medical News Today*, November 21, 2014, https://www.medicalnewstoday.com/articles/285917.
2. Jin-Soo Kim, Rebekah L. Wilson, Dennis R. Taaffe, Daniel A. Galvão, Elin Gray, and Robert U. Newton, "Myokine Expression and Tumor-Suppressive Effect of Serum after 12 wk of Exercise in Prostate Cancer Patients on ADT," *Medicine and Science in Sports and Exercise* 54, no. 2 (February 1, 2022): 197–205, https://pubmed.ncbi.nlm.nih.gov/34559721/.
3. Adi Narayan, "Is Running Bad for Your Knees? Maybe Not," *Time*, December 25, 2009, https://content.time.com/time/health/article/0,8599,1948208,00.html.
4. Erin Digitale, "Running Slows the Aging Clock, Stanford Researchers Find," *Stanford Medicine News*, August 11, 2008, https://med.stanford.edu/news/all-news/2008/08/running-slows-the-aging-clock-stanford-researchers-find.html.
5. Joey SJ Smeets et al., "Protein Synthesis Rates of Muscle, Tendon, Ligament, Cartilage, and Bone Tissue in Vivo in Humans," *PLOS One* 14, no. 11 (November 7, 2019), doi:10.1371/journal.pone.0224745.
6. Dan Brennan, "The Difference between Walking and Running," *WebMD*, November 15, 2021, https://www.webmd.com/fitness-exercise/difference-between-walking-and-running.
7. Maren S. Fragala et al., "Resistance Training for Older Adults: Position Statement from the National Strength and Conditioning Association," *Journal of Strength and Conditioning Research* 33, no. 8 (August 2019): 2019–52, doi:10.1519/JSC.0000000000003230.
8. Scott H. Hogan, *Built from Broken: A Science-Based Guide to Healing Painful Joints, Preventing Injuries, and Rebuilding Your Body* (Palm Beach Gardens, FL: SaltWrap, 2021).

Chapter Seven

1. Melinda Parrish, "Time to Defund the Diet Industry?" *HuffPost*, March 10, 2017, https://www.huffpost.com/entry/time-to-defund-the-diet-industry_b_58c2b63ee4b0c3276fb783c7.

Chapter Eight

1. Alejandro Gómez-Bruton, Alejandro Gónzalez-Agüero, Alba Gómez-Cabello, José A. Casajús, and Germán Vicente-Rodríguez, "Is Bone Tissue Really Affected by Swimming? A Systematic Review," *PLOS One* 8, no. 8 (August 2013), doi:10.1371/journal.pone.0070119.

Chapter Nine

1. The League of American Bicyclists, "About Smart Cycling," accessed July 5, 2023, https://bikeleague.org/ridesmart/.

Chapter Ten

1. Kenneth Cooper, *Aerobics* (New York: Bantam Books, 1968).
2. Gretchen Reynolds, "Is It Better to Work Out in the Morning or at Night?" *Washington Post*, September 21, 2022, https://www.washingtonpost.com/wellness/2022/09/21/best-time-exercise-workout-men-women/.
3. Eleftherios A. Makris, Pasha Hadidi, and Kyriacos A. Athanasiou, "The Knee Meniscus: Structure-Function, Pathophysiology, Current Repair Techniques, and Prospects for Regeneration," *Biomaterials* 32, no. 30 (July 18, 2011): 7411–31, doi:10.1016/j.biomaterials.2011.06.037.
4. Grace H. Lo et al., "Running Does Not Increase Symptoms or Structural Progression in People with Knee Osteoarthritis: Data from the Osteoarthritis Initiative," *Clinical Rheumatology* 37, no. 9 (May 4, 2018): 2497–504, doi:10.1007/s10067-018-4121-3.
5. N. Glass et al., "Examining Sex Differences in Knee Pain: The Multicenter Osteoarthritis Study," *Osteoarthritis Cartilage* 22, no. 8 (July 4, 2014): 1100–106, doi:10.1016/j.joca.2014.06.030.
6. VO Onywera, FK Kiplamai, MK Boit, and YP Pitsiladis, "Food and Macronutrient Intake of Elite Kenyan Distance Runners," *International Journal of Sport Nutrition and Exercise Metabolism* 14, no. 6 (December 2004): 709–19, doi:10.1123/ijsnem.14.6.709.

Chapter Twelve

1. Stephanie Winston, *Getting Organized* (New York: Grand Central Publishing, 1991).
2. CareerTrack, *How to Organize Your Life and Get Rid of Clutter* (New York: CareerTrack, 2006).
3. National Institute on Aging, "How Can Strength Training Build Healthier Bodies as We Age?" *Research Highlights*, June 30, 2022, https://www.nia.nih.gov/news/how-can-strength-training-build-healthier-bodies-we-age.
4. Jay M. Hoffman, *Hunza: 15 Secrets of the World's Healthiest and Oldest Living People* (Valley Center, CA: Professional Press Publishing, 1985).

Chapter Fourteen

1. Jacob Hunnicutt, Ka He, and Pengcheng Xun, "Dietary Iron Intake and Body Iron Stores Are Associated with Risk of Coronary Heart Disease in a

Meta-Analysis of Prospective Cohort Studies," *The Journal of Nutrition* 144, no. 3 (March 2014): 359–66, doi:10.3945/jn.113.185124.

2. John McDougall, *McDougall's Medicine: A Challenging Second Opinion* (Piscataway, NJ: New Century Publishers, 1985), 231–49.

3. J. Kjeldsen-Dragh et al., "Controlled Trial of Testing and One-Year Vegetarian Diet in Rheumatoid Arthritis," *The Lancet* 338, no. 8772 (October 12, 1991): 899–902, doi:10.1016/0140-6736(91)91770-u.

4. Kenneth Cooper, *Aerobics* (New York: Bantam Books, 1968), 4–5.

Chapter Fifteen

1. AL Klatsky, GD Friedman, and MA Armstrong, "Coffee Use Prior to Myocardial Infarction Restudied: Heavier Intake May Increase the Risk," *American Journal of Epidemiology* 132, no. 3 (September 1990): 479–88, doi:10.1093/oxfordjournals.aje.a115684.

2. DP Kiel, DT Felson, MT Hannan, JJ Anderson, and PW Wilson, "Caffeine and the Risk of Hip Fracture: The Framingham Study," *American Journal of Epidemiology* 132, no. 4 (October 1990): 675–84, doi:10.1093/oxfordjournals. aje.a115709.

3. Li Chen, Ruiyi Liu, Yong Zhao, and Zumin Shi, "High Consumption of Soft Drinks Is Associated with an Increased Risk of Fracture: A 7-Year Follow-Up Study," *Nutrients* 12, no. 2 (February 2020): 530, doi:10.3390/nu12020530.

4. Jennifer Huber, "Christopher Gardner Busts Myths about Milk," *Stanford Medicine News Center*, August 17, 2018, https://med.stanford.edu/news/all-news/2018/08/christopher-gardner-busts-myths-about-milk.html.

5. AG Marsh, TV Sanchez, O. Midkelsen, J. Keiser, and G. Mayor, "Cortical Bone Density of Adult Lacto-Ovo-Vegetarian and Omnivorous Women," *Journal of the American Dietetic Association* 76, no. 2 (1980): 148–51, PMID: 7391450.

6. Daniel Leigey, James Irrgang, Kimberly Francis, Peter Cohen, and Vonda Wright, "Participation in High-Impact Sports Predicts Bone Mineral Density in Senior Olympic Athletes," *Sports Health* 1, no. 6 (November 2009): 508–13, doi:10.1177/1941738109347979.

7. US Food and Drug Administration, "FDA Drug Safety Communication: Safety Update for Osteoporosis Drugs, Bisphosphonates, and Atypical Fractures," last modified February 6, 2018, https://www.fda.gov/drugs/drug-safety-and-availability/fda-drug-safety-communication-safety-update-osteoporosis-drugs-bisphosphonates-and-atypical.

8. BE Nordin and RP Heaney, "Calcium Supplementation of the Diet: Justified by Present Evidence," *British Medical Journal* 300 (April 1990): 1056–60, doi:10.1136/bmj.300.6731.1056.

9. RB Mazess and W. Mather, "Bone Mineral Content of North Alaskan Eskimos," *The American Journal of Clinical Nutrition* 27, no. 9 (September 1974): 916–25, doi:10.1093/ajcn/27.8.916.

10. Virginia Messina and Mark Messina, *The Vegetarian Way: Total Health for You and Your Family* (New York: Crown, 1996).

11. PC Rambaut and AW Goode, "Skeletal Changes during Space Flight," *Lancet* 2, no. 8463 (November 9, 1985): 1050–2, doi:10.1016/s0140-6736(85)90916-x.

12. JA Monro, R. Leon, and BK Puri, "The Risk of Lead Contamination in Bone Broth Diets," *Medical Hypotheses* 80, no. 4 (April 2013): 389–90, doi:10.1016/j.mehy.2012.12.026.

13. Daniel Wadsworth and Sally Lark, "Effects of Whole-Body Vibration Training on the Physical Function of the Frail Elderly: An Open, Randomized Controlled Trial," *Archives of Physical Medicine and Rehabilitation* 101, no. 7 (July 2020): 1111–9, doi:10.1016/j.apmr.2020.02.009.

14. Everett B. Lohman III, Jerrold Scott Petrofsky, Colleen Maloney-Hinds, Holly Betts-Schwab, and Donna Thorpe, "The Effect of Whole Body Vibration on Lower Extremity Skin Blood Flow in Normal Subjects," *Medical Science Monitor: International Medical Journal of Experimental and Clinical Research* 13, no. 2 (February 2007): CR71–6, PMID: 17261985.

15. William J. Kraemer and Nicholas A. Ratamess, "Hormonal Responses and Adaptations to Resistance Exercise and Training," *Sports Medicine* 35, no. 4 (2005): 339–61, doi:10.2165/00007256-200535040-00004.

Chapter Sixteen

1. Kent C. Holtzmuller, personal communication, July 1990.

Chapter Seventeen

1. Louie Psihoyos, dir., *The Game Changers* (ReFuel Productions, 2018), https://www.netflix.com/watch/81157840.

2. T. Hirayama, "Epidemiology of Prostate Cancer with Special Reference to the Role of Diet," *National Cancer Institute Monograph* 53 (November 1979): 149–55, PMID: 537622.

3. John R. Lee, *Natural Progesterone: The Multiple Roles of a Remarkable Hormone* (RLL Publishing, 1995).

4. Ibid.

5. Vanadin Seifert-Klauss and Jerilynn C. Prior, "Progesterone and Bone: Actions Promoting Bone Health in Women," *Journal of Osteoporosis* (October 31, 2010): 845180, doi:10.4061/2010/845180.

6. M. Oettel and AK Mukhopadhyay, "Progesterone: The Forgotten Hormone in Men?" *The Aging Male* 7, no. 3 (September 2004): 236–57, doi:10.1080/13685530400004199.

7. John McDougall and Mary McDougall, *The McDougall Program for Women* (New York: Plume, 2000).

8. Ibid.

9. Robin Marantz Henig, *How a Woman Ages* (New York: Ballantine Books, 1985).

10. Phillip Whitten, *The Complete Book of Swimming* (New York: Random House, 1994).

11. JA Mares-Perlman, "Contribution of Epidemiology to Understanding Relations of Diet to Age-Related Cataract," *The American Journal of Clinical Nutrition* 66, no. 4 (1997): 739–40, doi:10.1093/ajcn/66.4.739.

12. ST Mayne, "Beta-Carotene, Carotenoids, and Disease Prevention in Humans," *FASEB Journal* 10, no. 7 (1996): 690–701, PMID: 8635686.

13. Shivam Joshi, Sean Hashmi, Sanjeev Shah, and Kamyar Kalantar-Zadeh, "Plant-Based Diets for Prevention and Management of Chronic Kidney Disease," *Current Opinion in Nephrology and Hypertension* 29, no. 1 (2020): 16–21, doi:10.1097/MNH.0000000000000574.

14. National Institute on Alcohol Abuse and Alcoholism, "Alcohol's Effects on the Body," https://www.niaaa.nih.gov/alcohols-effects-health/alcohols-effects-body.

Chapter Eighteen

1. SVS Meldpunt Klachten Siliconen, "Prof. JW Cohen Tervaert FDA Meeting Breast Implants March 25th 2019," uploaded March 27, 2019, YouTube video, 24:15, https://www.youtube.com/watch?v=3QwMOoHhPKw.

2. Roger Wixtrom et al., "Heavy Metals in Breast Implant Capsules and Breast Tissue: Findings from the Systemic Symptoms in Women-Biospecimen Analysis Study: Part 2," *Aesthetic Surgery Journal* 42, no. 9 (August 24, 2022): 1067–76, doi:10.1093/asj/sjac106.

3. Hong Cheng, Bobo Yang, Tao Ke, Shaojun Li, Xiaobo Yang, Michael Aschner, and Pan Chen, "Mechanisms of Metal-Induced Mitochondrial Dysfunction in Neurological Disorders," *Toxics* 9, no. 6 (June 2021): 142, doi:10.3390/toxics9060142.

4. Ibid.

5. Agency for Toxic Substances and Disease Registry, "What Are the Physiologic Effects of Arsenic Exposure?" last modified May 19, 2023, https://www.atsdr.cdc.gov/csem/arsenic/physiologic_effects.html#.

6. Brooke Goldner, *Goodbye Lupus: How a Medical Doctor Healed Herself Naturally with Supermarket Foods* (Austin, TX: CreateSpace Independent Publishing, 2015).

Chapter Twenty

1. KK Carroll, "Experimental Evidence of Dietary Factors and Hormone-Dependent Cancers," *Cancer Research* 35, no. 11 pt. 2 (November 1975): 3374–83, PMID: 1104150.

2. AB Lowenthals and ME Anderson, "Diet and Cancer," *Cancer* 39, no. 4 (April 1977): 1809–14, doi:10.1002/1097-0142(197704)39:4+<1809::aid-cncr2820390811>3.0.co;2-o.

3. EL Wynder, T. Kajitani, J. Kuno, JC Lucas Jr., A. Depalo, and J. Farrow, "A Comparison of Survival Rates between American and Japanese Patients with Breast Cancer," *Surgery, Gynecology and Obstetrics* 117 (August 1963): 196–200, PMID: 14048012.

4. "Clinical Implications of Surgeon General's Report on Smoking and Health," *Journal of the National Medical Association* 71 (July 1979): 713–5.

5. O. Carl Simonton, Stephanie Matthews-Simonton, and James L. Creighton, *Getting Well Again: The Bestselling Classic about the Simontons' Revolutionary Lifesaving Self-Awareness Techniques* (New York: Bantam, 1992).

6. Stacy Simon, "How Exercise Can Lower Cancer Risk," *American Cancer Society*, February 19, 2020, https://www.cancer.org/cancer/latest-news/how-exercise-can-lower-cancer-risk.html.

7. HW Kohl, RE LaPorte, and SN Blair, "Physical Activity and Cancer: An Epidemiological Perspective," *Sports Medicine* 6, no. 4 (October 1988): 222–37, doi:10.2165/00007256-198806040-00004.

8. CB Mueller, F. Ames, and GD Anderson, "Breast Cancer in 3558 Women: Age as a Significant Determinant in the Rate of Dying and Causes of Death," *Surgery* 83, no. 2 (February 1978): 123–32, PMID: 622685.

9. Rowan T. Chlebowski et al., "Association of Low-Fat Dietary Pattern with Breast Cancer Overall Survival," *JAMA Oncology* 4, no. 10 (October 2018): e181212, doi:10.1001/jamaoncol.2018.1212.

Resources

Books

Bailey, Covert. *The Ultimate Fit or Fat.* Boston: Rux Martin/Houghton Mifflin Harcourt, 2000.

Barnard, Neal D. *Foods That Fight Pain: Proven Dietary Solutions for Maximum Pain Relief without Drugs.* Emmaus, PA: Rodale, 2008.

———. *Food for Life: How the New Four Food Groups Can Save Your Life.* New York: Harmony Books, 1994.

———. *The Power of Your Plate: A Plan for Better Living.* Summertown, TN: Book Publishing Company, 1995.

Borysewicz, Edward. *Bicycle Road Racing: The Complete Program for Training and Competition.* Brattleboro, VT: Velo-News Corp, 1985.

Cooper, Kenneth. *Aerobics.* New York: Bantam Books, 1968.

Harris, William. *The Scientific Basis of Vegetarianism.* Honolulu: Hawaii Health Publishers, 1995.

Henig, Robin Marantz. *How a Woman Ages.* New York: Ballantine Books, 1985.

Keon, Joseph. *The Truth about Breast Cancer: A 7-Step Prevention Plan.* Mill Valley, CA: Parissound Publishing, 1999.

Klaper, Michael. *Vegan Nutrition: Pure and Simple.* Umatilla, FL: Gentle World, 1987.

Kradjian, Robert M. *Save Yourself from Breast Cancer: Life Choices That Can Help You Reduce the Odds.* New York: Berkley Publishing, 1994.

Lee, John. *Natural Progesterone: The Multiple Roles of a Remarkable Hormone.* Sebastopol, CA: BLL Publishing, 2000.

McDougall, John. *The McDougall Program: 12 Days to Dynamic Health.* New York: Plume, 1991.

———. *McDougall's Medicine: A Challenging Second Opinion.* Clinton, NJ: New Win Publishing, 1986.

———. *The McDougall Program for Maximum Weight Loss.* New York: Penguin Publishing Group, 1995.

McDougall, John and Mary McDougall. *The McDougall Program for Women: What Every Woman Needs to Know to Be Healthy for Life.* New York: Dutton, 1998.

———. *The McDougall Plan.* Clinton, NJ: New Win Publishing, 1985.

———. *The McDougall Program for a Healthy Heart: A Life-Saving Approach to Preventing and Treating Heart Disease*. New York: Plume, 1998.

———. *The New McDougall Cookbook: 300 Delicious Low-Fat, Plant-Based Recipes*. New York: Plume, 1997.

McDougall, Mary. *The McDougall Health-Supporting Cookbook*. vols. 1–2. Clinton, NJ: New Win Publishing, 1985, 1986.

Morra, Marion and Eve Potts. *Choices: Realistic Alternatives in Cancer Treatment*. New York: Avon, 1994.

Notelovitz, Morris. *Stand Tall! Every Woman's Guide to Preventing and Treating Osteoporosis*. Gainesville, FL: Triad Publishing, 1998.

Ornish, Dean. *Dr. Dean Ornish's Program for Reversing Heart Disease*. New York: Ovy Books, 1995.

———. *Eat More, Weigh Less: Dr. Dean Ornish's Life Choice Program for Losing Weight Safely While Eating Abundantly*. New York: William Morrow, 2002.

Ostrander, Sheila and Lynn Schroeder. *Super-Learning*. Miller Place, NY: Laurel Publications, 1982.

Prins, Jan. *The Illustrated Swimmer*. Honolulu, HI: He'e, 1982.

Robbins, John. *Diet for a New America: How Your Food Choices Affect Your Health, Your Happiness, and the Future of Life on Earth*. Tiburon, CA: HJ Kramer, 2012.

———. *May All Be Fed: A Diet for a New World*. New York: Avon, 1993.

———. *Reclaiming Our Health: Exploding the Medical Myth and Embracing the Sources of True Healing*. Tiburon, CA: HJ Kramer, 1996.

Scott, Dave. *Dave Scott's Triathlon Training*. New York: Touchstone, 1986.

Siegel, Bernie. *Love, Medicine and Miracles: Lessons Learned about Self-Healing from a Surgeon's Experience with Exceptional Patients*. New York: William Morrow, 2011.

Simonton, O. Carl, Stephanie Matthews-Simonton, and James L. Creighton. *Getting Well Again: The Bestselling Classic about the Simontons' Revolutionary Lifesaving Self-Awareness Techniques*. New York: Bantam, 1992.

Organizations and Periodicals

American Cancer Society Reach to Recovery program, 3380 Chastain Meadows Parkway NW, Suite 200, Kennesaw, GA 30144. Website: https://reach.cancer.org/.

American Vegan Society, 56 Danish Lane, PO Box 369, Malaga, NJ 08328. Website: https://americanvegan.org/.

Bicycling, 400 South Tenth Street, Emmaus, PA 18098. Website: https://www.bicycling.com/.

Smart Cycling, The League of American Bicyclists, 1612 K Street NW, Suite 1102, Washington, DC 20006. Tel.: 202-822-1333. Website: https://bikeleague.org/ridesmart/.

Ruth Heidrich's website: https://ruthheidrich.com/.

International Vegetarian Union. Website: https://ivu.org/north-america.html.

Dr. McDougall's Health and Medical Center, PO Box 14039, Santa Rosa, CA 95402. Email: office@drmcdougall.com. Website: https://www.drmcdougall.com/.

A Race for Life video and *The Race for Life Cookbook*, 1415 Victoria Street #1106, Honolulu, HI 96822.

Road Runners Club of America national office, 1501 Langston Boulevard, Suite 140, Arlington, VA 22209. Tel.: 703-525-3890. Website: https://www.rrca.org/.

Runner's World, Hearst Magazines, Inc., 300 W 57th Street, New York, NY 10019-3779. Website: https://www.runnersworld.com/.

Running Network LLC. Website: https://www.runningnetwork.com/.

Swim Magazine, GMC Publications Ltd., 86 High Street, Lewes, BN7 1XU, United Kingdom. Website: https://justswimmag.com/.

Vegan Outreach, 3053 Freeport Boulevard #282, Sacramento, CA 95818. Tel.: 530-207-0119. Website: https://veganoutreach.org/.

Vegetarian Resource Group, PO Box 1463, Baltimore, MD 21203. Tel.: 410-366-8343.

Website: https://www.vrg.org/.

Vegetarian Times, Outside, Inc., 1600 Pearl Street, Boulder, CO 80302. Tel.: 855-OUT-0567. Website: https://www.vegetariantimes.com/.

Seven-Day Meal Plan (*see recipes)

MONDAY
Breakfast: Oatmeal with Sliced Banana
Lunch: Pho* (Vietnamese Soup)
Dinner: Baked Okinawan Purple Potatoes with Veggies

TUESDAY
Breakfast: Buckwheat Cereal with Orange Slices
Lunch: Vegan Sandwich*
Dinner: Spaghetti Marinara with Tossed Green Salad

WEDNESDAY
Breakfast: Wheat Berries with Sliced Mango
Lunch: Texas Fries*, Apple and Pear Slices
Dinner: Pizza*

THURSDAY
Breakfast: Millet with Sliced Apples
Lunch: Fruit Sandwich*
Dinner: Baked Squash with Brown Rice and Broccoli

FRIDAY
Breakfast: Shredded Wheat with Pineapple Chunks
Lunch: Split Pea Soup*
Dinner: Lentil Loaf* with Corn on the Cob

SATURDAY
Breakfast: Pancakes with Blueberries*
Lunch: Baked Potato with Salsa
Dinner: Wild Rice with Beets and Brussel Sprouts

SUNDAY
Breakfast: Waffles with Strawberries*
Lunch: Stuffed Pita Bread Sandwich
Dinner: Eggplant Szechwan with Brown Rice*

Recipes

Two-Minute Oatmeal

    1/2 cup organic old-fashioned rolled oats
    1 banana
    1 tsp blackstrap molasses

Pour oats into cereal bowl and add water to cover. Microwave for 3 minutes. Add molasses and sliced banana or any combination of fruit.

Pho (Vietnamese Soup)

    1 cup cooked brown rice
    1 small package nori (seaweed)
    1/2 bunch chopped parsley
    1 tbsp miso
    1–2 cups water (to top off bowl)
    1/2 tsp hot chili sauce (to taste)
    1/2 bunch beet greens, cabbage, or other greens

Add all ingredients to large soup bowl and microwave for 4 minutes. Stir thoroughly.

Rice Ramen Curry

    1 pot cooked brown rice
    1 cup chopped cilantro
    1 package low-fat ramen noodles
    1 tbsp curry powder
    1/2 cup raisins

Break up ramen noodles while still in package with the heel of the hand until there are no large chunks. Open package, remove spice packet, and mix crushed noodles with freshly cooked brown rice. (The heat of the rice "cooks" the noodles.) Add the spice packet, curry powder, parsley, and raisins. Ready to serve hot or cold.

Vegan Sandwich

    Assorted sliced veggies, e.g., Romaine lettuce, kale, tomato, cucumber, sprouts

    2 slices whole-grain bread or 1 pita bread

Arrange sliced veggies between slices of bread or in pita pocket. Add condiments if desired.

Wheat Berries

Cook wheat berries on stovetop until soft. Alternatively, pour wheat berries into a thermos of boiling water, cover, and let sit overnight. Add fruit and serve. This technique works with all types of whole grains.

Texas Fries

    2–3 large potatoes, any type

Cut into quarters lengthwise and microwave approximately 7 to 10 minutes, depending on size. They taste great just plain, but you can sprinkle vinegar, garlic powder, and paprika or any other combination of herbs and spices on them.

Pizza

    1 pita bread

    1 tbsp oregano

    1 can tomato sauce or 1/2 cup salsa

    1 tbsp basil

    Veggies, e.g., sliced bell pepper, mushrooms, chopped onions, sprouts

Spread veggies on split pita bread. Bake or microwave until bubbly. For a cheesy topping, sprinkle on some nutritional yeast.

Fruit Sandwich

    Assorted fruits

    Pita or other whole-grain bread

Arrange slices of fruit in pita pocket or on bread slices.

Split Pea Soup

    2 cups split peas
    1 onion, chopped
    2 quarts water
    1 pinch cayenne
    4 ribs celery, diced
    1 bay leaf
    2 carrots, diced
    1/2 tsp thyme

Combine all ingredients in a large pot, bring to a boil and simmer 1 hour, or cook 4 hours in a slow cooker.

Lentil Loaf

    2 cups cooked lentils
    1 can tomato sauce
    1 onion, chopped
    1 cup organic rolled oats, uncooked
    Herbs, e.g., garlic, parsley, basil, oregano, fennel

Preheat oven to 350 degrees Fahrenheit. Combine all ingredients, mixing well. Put into 8×4×2 in loaf pan. Bake 45 minutes.

Pancakes or Waffles

    2 cups whole-wheat flour
    1 tbsp blackstrap molasses
    1 cup organic rolled oats
    1 tbsp baking powder
    3 cups water
    1 tbsp vanilla
    1 tbsp cinnamon

Combine ingredients in a medium bowl, taking care not to over-mix. Turn griddle on medium high for about 5 minutes or until a drop of water dances on the surface. Alternatively, turn on waffle iron for about 10 minutes. Spray surface with non-stick cooking spray. Ladle batter onto griddle or iron. Turn pancakes when bubbles appear and give them another minute or so. Waffle is ready when steam stops rising, after about a minute and a half. Do not open the waffle iron too soon or the waffle will separate. Use desired fruity topping such as berries, preserve, or applesauce.

Eggplant Szechwan

  2–3 eggplants
  2 tbsp low-sodium soy sauce
  1 green onion, sliced
  1 tbsp cornstarch
  1 tsp chili sauce, or to taste
  2 cups water
  1 tbsp ginger, minced and preferably fresh

Slice eggplants. Put in a large, round casserole dish. Add cornstarch to the water, mixing well. Add mixture along with the remaining ingredients to eggplant and bake. Alternatively, bake in microwave for about 5 to 6 minutes or in conventional oven for about 25 minutes at 350 degrees Fahrenheit.

Interpretation of Laboratory Tests

The following information, sourced from different laboratories, is provided as a rough guide to help you understand the results of your lab tests. Since there are variations between laboratories, accuracy is not guaranteed. Use this appendix to learn more about what lab tests tell you about your body. The figures in parentheses represent the ideal ranges. Measurement abbreviations are as follows: mg (milligram), mm (millimeter), dL (deciliter or a tenth of a liter), μL (microliter or one millionth of a liter), mEq (milliequivalent or one-thousandth of an equivalent), mcg (microgram or one millionth of a gram), ng (nanogram or one billionth of a gram), μmol (also umol) (micromole or one millionth of the molecular weight).

CHOL (100–160 mg/dL): This stands for blood cholesterol and is probably the most important figure. If you have an average blood cholesterol level (220 mg/dL), then you have an average risk for heart attack (more than 50 percent), breast cancer (12.5 percent for women), colon cancer (5 percent), and gallbladder disease (20 percent). Cholesterol is found only in animal products, and all animal products contain cholesterol. Your own body makes all the cholesterol you need. When you eat additional cholesterol in the form of animal products, it is readily absorbed, but your liver can break down only a limited amount of this substance per day. The excess accumulates in body tissues such as arteries, skin, organs, and body fat. Your blood cholesterol level reflects the level of cholesterol in your body. The ideal level is 150 mg/dl or less. For most people, replacing animal foods with starches, vegetables, and fruits will cause their cholesterol to fall by 30–100 mg/dL in fewer than three weeks. Maintenance of this diet will result in continued improvement. Excreted cholesterol enters the gallbladder, thereby contributing to gallstones (90 percent of which are made of cholesterol). Cholesterol in the colon is believed to be involved in colon cancer. A change to a no-cholesterol diet is the most effective and safest way to lower your cholesterol. No plant food contains any cholesterol as plants' cell walls are made from fiber. Note, however, that coconuts and chocolate contain enough saturated fat to raise cholesterol levels in the blood.

HDL (male 26–66 mg/dL; female 30–75 mg/dL): This stands for high-density lipoprotein, a fraction of the total cholesterol level with some predictive value for risk of heart disease. HDL is an end product of cholesterol metabolism and represents the cholesterol that is leaving body tissues and on its way to being excreted by the liver. If your level is low and you're consuming the SAD diet, you should consider this as an indication that it's time to start a low- to no-cholesterol diet. People on low-cholesterol diets have lower HDL because of their low total cholesterol.

GLUCOSE (65–120 mg/dL): This indicates the sugar in your blood. When you haven't eaten for a while, your glucose level is normally between 65 and 120 mg/dL. When the body loses control of sugar levels, the condition is called diabetes (indicated by glucose levels over 120 mg/dL). Most cases of diabetes (95 percent) fall under type 2 diabetes (so-called adult-onset diabetes) and are caused by a high-fat, low-fiber diet. Dietary correction will therefore solve the problem for most people. Exercise and weight loss also help. Type 1 or childhood-onset diabetes is a different condition that results from the destruction of portions of the pancreas that produce insulin. While a proper diet will not cure this type of diabetes, it will still certainly help. Hypoglycemia is the condition of low blood sugar (below 50 mg/dl). Another test (the five-hour glucose-tolerance test) is used to make a diagnosis. The cause and correction are also diet-related.

A1C or HbA1C (below 5.7 normal; 5.7-6.4 pre-diabetic; 6.5 or above diabetic): This number gives an average blood-sugar reading for the past three months.

CRP or Sed Rate (normal values range from less than 10 to less than 30 mm/hour, depending on age and gender): These tests measure inflammation markers in the body.

BUN (6–25 mg/dL): This stands for blood urea nitrogen, the breakdown product of protein. BUN is made in the liver and excreted by the kidneys. Low-protein diets lower BUN levels. Kidney disease can cause BUN levels to rise and make people feel ill.

CREA (0.7–1.4 mg/dL): This stands for creatinine, a breakdown product from muscle that is excreted by the kidneys. Elevated levels usually mean kidney disease.

URIC ACID (2.2–7.7 mg/dL): This is a breakdown product of purines, which are found in high-protein foods such as meat (including chicken and seafood), cheese, and beans. Large amounts of uric acid can lead to gout (arthritis) and kidney stones.

TRIG (50–275 mg/dL): This stands for triglycerides, or blood fats. If your blood were to sit in a test tube overnight, fat would rise to form a layer at the top. High levels are associated with heart attack, diabetes, and poor circulation, which result in chest pain, leg pain, and fatigue. Your triglycerides are elevated when you consume fats, simple sugars, and alcoholic beverages. Even fruit and fruit juice can elevate triglycerides levels in sensitive people. Exercise, high-fiber foods, and weight loss will lower triglycerides to healthy levels. Note that sometimes, during a period of weight loss, triglycerides may temporarily rise due to the movement of fat from fat tissues to the blood. You should try to keep your levels below 200 mg/dL.

BILI (1.1–1.7 mg/dL): This is a breakdown product of red blood cells. It is therefore elevated when there is a lot of breakdown of blood cells or when the liver is diseased and unable to adequately excrete it. Many people show a slight elevation (up to 3 mg/dL) that may occur as a result of overnight fasting. The best indication of normal liver function is that all the other liver tests give normal results.

SGOT (7–50 µl), SGPT (7–50 µl), LDH (90–225 µl): These are abbreviations for liver enzymes that are released when the liver is injured. Gallbladder disease, excess alcohol consumption, and viruses causing hepatitis are the most common causes of elevation.

ALK PHOS (30–115 µl): This stands for alkaline phosphatase, an enzyme from either bones or the liver. Levels can be elevated in bone or gallbladder disease.

INORG P (2.0–4.7 mg/dL): This stands for inorganic phosphorus. Levels increase with more phosphorus in your diet.

CALCIUM (8.8–10.8 mg/dL): This mineral has many functions in the body. Calcium in the blood must be kept at minimum critical levels. Therefore, this number is almost always normal. Abnormal values usually reflect a laboratory error or a decrease in albumin protein in the blood due to liver or kidney disease. The level of calcium in your blood does not reflect the amount of calcium in your diet or in your bones.

NA (135–145 mEq/L): This is sodium, a mineral found in large quantities in the body. Its level does not reflect dietary intake of salt. Sometimes, sodium level is low if you are taking diuretics or medications to lower blood pressure.

K (3.5–5.5 mEq/L): This is potassium, a mineral also found in large amounts in the body. Its level does not reflect dietary intake except in the case of serious kidney disease. Potassium level can be low if you are on diuretics. This mineral must be kept in the normal range or death can result.

CL (96–110 mEq/L) and CO2 (25–32 mEq/L): These stand for chlorine and carbon dioxide, which are usually at normal levels in the blood unless you are on certain medications.

TOT PRO (6.2–8.3 g/dL): This represents the amount of total protein floating in the blood. Proteins are made primarily by the liver and the immune system. They may be elevated in the case of certain infections and disease of the bone marrow.

ALBUMIN (3.6–5.2 g/dL): This is a protein made in the liver. Its level goes down with serious liver and kidney disease.

GLOBULIN (2.5 g/dL): This is the protein made by the immune system for defense.

A/G (1.1–2.2): This stands for the ratio of albumin to globulin.

HEMOGLOBIN (male 14–18 g/dL; female 12–16 g/dL): This is the oxygen-carrying, red-pigmented, iron-containing substance in the blood. Hemoglobin levels reflect the number of red blood cells in the body, and a low level can mean anemia. In the US, 20 percent of women have iron-deficiency anemia. Dairy products contribute to this problem in several ways. Cow's milk is deficient in iron, and the calcium and phosphorus in cow's milk complex iron from other sources, thus preventing its absorption. The fats in dairy products and other high-fat foods also cause higher levels of estrogen in women, resulting in heavier menstrual periods and more blood loss each month. Anyone with anemia should be checked for blood loss in their stools at the minimum.

HCT (40–55 percent, slightly lower in women): HCT or hematocrit shows the percentage of blood cells (mostly red blood cells) comprising the total blood volume. It is used as a test for anemia and dehydration, as well as to follow the course of therapy for anemia.

TIBC (200–400 mcg/100 mL): This stands for total iron-binding capacity, which is usually increased only with iron-deficiency anemia, a type of anemia associated with blood loss.

SERUM FERRITIN (30 mg/100 mL and up): This is a measure of the iron stores in the body. Decreased ferritin is found with iron deficiency but not with anemia of infection. Increased ferritin is found with excessive iron intake.

HOMOCYSTEINE (5–15 *μmol*/L): This is an amino acid associated with vascular disease.

GLOSSARY

Aerobic Integrity: The level of oxygen-burning exercise at which the body can produce a sustained output for an extended period of time without going into oxygen debt.

Amnesia: Lack or loss of memory. **Anterograde a.:** Loss of memory for events that occurred after the onset of the disease. **Retrograde a.:** Loss of memory for events that occurred before the onset of the disease.

Anaerobic: An inability to maintain an oxygen level in the body to support continued exercise, which leads to oxygen debt.

Anemia: The condition of deficient quantity or quality of the blood, usually marked by paleness and fatigue.

Angiogenesis: The formation of new blood vessels, which is necessary for both progress and spread of disease. This is the basis for the ability of cancerous cells to form their own blood supply, enabling them to travel to other parts of the body, typically the lungs, liver, bones, and brain, to set up new colonies of cancerous tumor. Angiogenesis occurs before the original tumor can grow to more than a few millimeters in size.

Areola: The pigmented area surrounding the nipple.

Biathlon: Any two-sport race, for example, a swim-run or a bike-run.

Biceps: The large flexor muscle of the front of the upper arm.

Biopsy: Examination of tissue removed from a living subject.

Carbohydrates: Compounds made up of carbon atoms in groups of six, plus hydrogen and oxygen atoms in proportions to form water. Carbohydrates have four calories per gram and are found primarily in starchy and sugary foods.

Chemotherapy: Treatment by powerful chemical compounds that have a toxic effect on specific cells or microorganisms. Cancer cells, which are frequently weak and disorganized, are usually more vulnerable to the effects of this treatment.

Cholesterol: A waxy substance produced in the liver of every animal. It makes up the structural integrity of all animal cells.

Endorphins: Chemicals produced by the body that create pleasant feelings. Endorphins contribute to the so-called "runner's high."

Epidemiology: The branch of science that studies the occurrence, distribution, and types of disease among populations.

Fascia: The band or sheet of connective tissue covering muscles.

Fat: The oily substance that covers the connective tissues of animals; an organic salt consisting of the glycerol radical C_3H_5 combined with a fatty acid. Fat has more than twice the number of calories of carbohydrates and protein—nine calories per gram.

Hydrostatic body-fat test: A method of estimating percentage of body fat by immersion in water.

Infiltrating ductal carcinoma: Moderately fast-metastasizing, invasive breast cancer accounting for about 65 percent of all breast cancer cases. It may spread to the liver, lungs, bones, and brain. It usually cannot be eradicated by local treatment of breast and lymph nodes and has spread to the bloodstream by the time clinical symptoms are evident.

Lacto-ovo-vegetarian: A person who avoids animal meat but still consumes dairy products and eggs. A lacto-ovo-vegetarian diet will still be high in animal fat and cholesterol, since milk has been referred to as "liquid meat."

LASIK (laser-assisted in situ keratomileusis): A procedure that corrects vision by changing the shape of the cornea. A hinged flap is cut on the surface of the cornea and a laser reshapes the underlying corneal tissue.

Lignans: An anti-cancer plant compound found in whole grains, cruciferous vegetables, sesame seeds, and flaxseeds.

Liposuction: A surgical procedure whereby fat is sucked out of the body in very specific areas.

Marathon: A footrace of 26.2 miles that originated in Greece in 490 BC. When the Athenians defeated the Persians, a messenger, Pheidippides, was sent to bear the news of the victory to Athens. The name is derived from the starting point of his run, the battle site of Marathon. Now, most cities and countries of the world conduct these races annually.

Mastectomy: The surgical amputation of the breast. **Modified radical m.:** Removal of the breast plus the skin, nipple, subcutaneous fat, fascia, and axillary (armpit) nodes. **Simple m.:** Removal of breast tissue only, leaving the skin and nipple. **Radical m.:** Removal of the breast, skin, nipple, fascia, subcutaneous fat, axillary nodes, and the pectoral (chest) muscles. **Lumpectomy:** Removal of the tumor and a margin of healthy surrounding tissue.

Metastasis: Spread of disease from one organ to another through angiogenesis.

Microbiome: The set of microorganisms in a particular environment, used most often to refer to the colon.

Myokines: Proteins produced in the body by exercise in the skeletal muscles that have suppressing effects on cancer.

Oncology, -ist: The study of tumors and cancers and the person who studies them.

Osteoporosis: The thinning or abnormal porousness of the bones, the cause of which is still debated. Most recent studies show that the best treatment, as well as prevention, for this condition involves exercise and a low-protein diet.

Phytoestrogens: Plant estrogens, which are weaker than normal estrogen and can actually bind to or block excess estrogen in the body rather than increase total estrogen levels.

Protein: Combinations of amino acids and their derivatives found in animal and vegetable tissues. Protein has four calories per gram.

Reconstructive breast surgery: The insertion of an implant under the chest skin or muscle to restore the normal body contours that were lost due to an amputated breast. Nipples and areolae may also be reconstructed using various body parts such as earlobes, skin from the upper inner thigh, and so on.

Sarcopenia: The loss of muscle, along with muscle strength, mobility, independence, psychological well-being, and quality of life, with aging.

Subcutaneous: Under the skin. May refer to implant placement in the context of reconstructive breast surgery, as opposed to sub-muscular, under the chest muscle.

Triathlon: Any three-sport race, conventionally a swim-bike-run.

Ultra-marathon: Any footrace longer than a marathon (26.2 miles).

Vegan: A philosophy and way of life including a diet that is devoid of all animal products, including seafood, dairy products, and eggs. Biochemically, there is very little difference between meat, dairy products, and eggs in terms of composition. All animal products are high in fat, high in cholesterol, low in iron, and completely lacking in fiber.

ABOUT THE AUTHOR

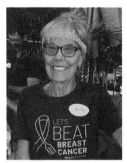 **Ruth Heidrich** received her PhD in Health Management in 1993 and is the author of *The Race For Life Cookbook*, *Senior Fitness*, and *Lifelong Running*. Diagnosed with an aggressive type of breast cancer in her mid-forties despite thinking she was extremely healthy having run marathons, she researched possible causes of breast cancer when exercise was not enough. She came upon Dr. John McDougall's research, which strongly indicated that the culprit was the Standard American Diet. This is a passionate example of how Ruth Heidrich turned tragedy into triumph using a medically sound diet and exercise program which has served her well for over forty years.

About the Publisher

Lantern Publishing & Media was founded in 2020 to follow and expand on the legacy of Lantern Books—a publishing company started in 1999 on the principles of living with a greater depth and commitment to the preservation of the natural world. Like its predecessor, Lantern Publishing & Media produces books on animal advocacy, veganism, religion, social justice, humane education, psychology, family therapy, and recovery. Lantern is dedicated to printing in the United States on recycled paper and saving resources in our day-to-day operations. Our titles are also available as ebooks and audiobooks.

To catch up on Lantern's publishing program, visit us at www.lanternpm.org.

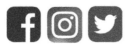

facebook.com/lanternpm
twitter.com/lanternpm
instagram.com/lanternpm